D0214709

HOW SCIENTISTS EXPLAIN DISEASE

HOW SCIENTISTS EXPLAIN DISEASE

Paul Thagard

PRINCETON UNIVERSITY PRESS   PRINCETON, NEW JERSEY

Copyright © 1999 by Princeton University Press
Published by Princeton University Press, 41 William Street,
Princeton, New Jersey 08540
In the United Kingdom: Princeton University Press,
Chichester, West Sussex
All Rights Reserved

Library of Congress Cataloging-in-Publication Data
Thagard, Paul.
How scientists explain disease / Paul Thagard.
p.   cm.
Includes bibliographical references and index.
ISBN 0-691-00261-4 (cloth : alk. paper)
1. Diseases—Causes and theories of causation.
2. Medicine—Research—Methodology.
3. Medicine—Philosophy.   4. Peptic ulcer—Etiology.
5. Helicobacter pylori infections.   I. Title.
RB151.T47   1999
616.07′1—dc21   98-34717   CIP

This book has been composed in Times Roman

The paper used in this publication meets the minimum requirements
of ANSI/NISO Z39.48-1992 (R1997) (*Permanence of Paper*)

http://pup.princeton.edu

Printed in the United States of America

1   3   5   7   9   10   8   6   4   2

_____ **For Adam, Daniel, and Ziva** _____

SANTÉ!

Contents

Figures

Tables

THIS BOOK is about the causes of disease and the causes of science. It is an attempt to answer the question: How do scientists learn about why people get sick? Explaining advances in medical science is similar to explaining diseases, in that both kinds of explanations require the assembly of complexes of interacting causes. Just as most diseases arise from the interaction of environmental and genetic factors, so medical theories arise from the interplay of psychological, physical, and social processes. I have written the book for two main audiences. The first consists of readers with a general interest in the development of medical knowledge about diseases such as peptic ulcer. The second consists of people studying the history, philosophy, psychology, or sociology of science, who will find here an investigation that combines and integrates all these approaches.

The case study at the core of this book is the development and acceptance of the theory that the primary cause of most peptic ulcers is infection by a recently discovered bacterium, *Helicobacter pylori*. I first encountered this case in 1993, when Dr. David Graham invited me to visit him at the Baylor College of Medicine in Houston. He had read my book *Conceptual Revolutions* and saw it as relevant to the rise of the bacterial theory of ulcers, which was first proposed in 1983 by two Australian physicians, Barry Marshall and Robin Warren. Initially, this theory was greeted with intense skepticism by medical experts, but by 1995 it had widespread support. Chapters 3 to 6 of this text provide an integrated explanation of these developments, discussing psychological processes of discovery and acceptance, physical processes involving instruments and experiments, and social processes of collaboration, communication, and consensus.

Chapters 1 and 2 set the stage for the ulcers case study by discussing the nature of explanations of scientific developments and of diseases, both of which are best described in terms of complex schemas that assemble multiple interacting causes. Chapter 1 presents explanation schemas that capture the main current approaches to the study of science, ranging from logical schemas favored by many philosophers to social schemas employed by sociologists. Chapter 2 reviews the most important medical explanation schemas in the history of medicine, from the Hippocratic theory of humors to very recent explanations based on molecular genetics. I argue that an integrated cognitive-social schema provides the most promising approach to explaining the growth of scientific knowledge, and chapters 3 to 6 fill out this schema in the case of the bacterial theory of ulcers.

Chapters 7 to 10 delve more deeply into cognitive mechanisms involving causality, analogy, and conceptual change. Chapter 7 discusses the meaning of the claim that bacteria cause ulcers and provides a general account of medical causal reasoning. Chapter 8 uses this account to explain why discovering the causes of diseases encounters many difficulties, which are illustrated by the development of ideas about scurvy, spongiform encephalopathies (e.g., mad cow disease), AIDS, and chronic fatigue syndrome. Analogical thinking has been important in many cases in the history of medicine that are described in chapter 9. Chapter 10 shows how the development of new medical theories can involve major kinds of conceptual change concerning diseases and their causes.

Chapters 11 to 13 investigate social processes that contribute to the growth of scientific knowledge. Collaboration was a major factor in the development and acceptance of the bacterial theory of ulcers, as it is in most current scientific work; chapter 11 provides a description and evaluation of this role. Chapter 12 describes a social process unique to medicine, the use of consensus conferences to reach authoritative conclusions that provide recommendations for medical practitioners. Increasingly, social interactions in science are being facilitated electronically by the various technologies available on the Internet, and chapter 13 discusses the contributions of these technologies to the development of scientific knowledge. In all three of these chapters, my concern is not only to describe social processes but also to evaluate their potential positive and negative effects on medical progress. Finally, chapter 14 uses ideas about distributed computing to portray science as a complex system of cognitive, social, and physical interactions. The book concludes with a defense of scientific rationality and realism.

Especially in chapter 13 but also in other chapters, I have referred to World Wide Web resources using universal resource locators beginning with "http." Web users can find live links for these references via my Web site at http://cogsci.uwaterloo.ca.

Acknowledgments

I OWE a great debt to medical researchers for very helpful conversations, and thank Drs. David Graham, Richard Hunt, Barry Marshall, J. Robin Warren, and Tadataka Yamada. Special thanks to David Graham for introducing me to the ulcers case and for providing feedback on my first attempts to understand it.

For research support I am very grateful to the Social Sciences and Humanities Research Council of Canada, the Natural Sciences and Engineering Research Council of Canada, and the Killam Fellowship program of the Canada Council. Thanks to Kim Honeyford and Kathleen Gorman for research assistance.

For various chapters of this book, I have adapted parts of previous articles, and I am grateful to the respective publishers for permission to reprint some of their contents:

Thagard, P. (1993). Societies of minds: Science as distributed computing. *Studies in History and Philosophy of Science*, *24*, 49–67. [Used in chapter 14.] Reprinted with permission of Elsevier Science.

Thagard, P. (1994). Mind, society, and the growth of knowledge. *Philosophy of Science*, *61*, 629–645. [Used in chapter 1.] Reprinted with permission of the University of Chicago Press.

Thagard, P. (1995). Explaining scientific change: Integrating the cognitive and the social. In D. Hull, M. Forbes, and R. Burian (Eds.), *PSA 1994*. Vol. 2 (pp. 298–303). East Lansing, MI: Philosophy of Science Association. [Used in chapter 1.] Reprinted with permission of the Philosophy of Science Association.

Thagard, P. (1996). The concept of disease: Structure and change. *Communication and Cognition*, *29*, 445–478. [Used in chapters 2 and 10.] Reprinted with permission of *Communication and Cognition*.

Thagard, P. (1997). Collaborative knowledge. *Noûs*, *31*, 242–261. [Used in chapter 11.] Reprinted with permission of Blackwell Publishers.

Thagard, P. (1997). Medical analogies: Why and how. In P. Langley and M. Shafto (Eds.), *Proceedings of the Nineteenth Annual Conference of the Cognitive Science Society* pp. 739–744. Mahway, N.J.: Erlbaum. [Used in chapter 9.] Reprinted with permission of the Cognitive Science Society.

Thagard, P. (1998). Explaining disease: Causes, correlations, and mechanisms. *Minds and Machines*, *8*, 61–78. [Used in chapter 7.] Reprinted with permission of Kluwer Academic Publisher.

Thagard, P. (1998). Ulcers and bacteria I: Discovery and acceptance. *Studies in History and Philosophy of Science. Part C. Studies in History and Philosophy of Biological and Biomedical Sciences*, 29, 107–136. [Used in chapters 3 and 4.] Reprinted with permission of Elsevier Science.

Thagard, P. (1998). Ulcers and bacteria II: Instruments, experiments, and social interactions. *Studies in History and Philosophy of Science. Part C. Studies in History and Philosophy of Biological and Biomedical Sciences*, 29, 317–342. [Used in chapters 5 and 6.] Reprinted with permission of Elsevier Science.

For assistance with particular articles, I am grateful to Kevin Dunbar, David Graham, Daniel Hausman, Ed Hutchins, Barry Marshall, Robert McCauley, Nancy Nersessian, Gary Olson, Paul Rusnock, Cameron Shelley, Herbert Simon, Miriam Solomon, and James van Evra. Thanks to Miriam Solomon and two anonymous referees for comments on a previous draft of the whole book, and to Sam Elworthy, Ziva Kunda, and Allison Aydelotte for useful suggestions.

Part One

EXPLANATIONS

CHAPTER 1

Explaining Science

IN THE 1950s, a doctor whose patient was diagnosed with a stomach ulcer would typically recommend that the patient relax and drink lots of milk. By the late 1970s, however, treatment had changed, and the doctor would probably prescribe Tagamet or one of the other acid-blocking drugs that had been developed. Today, in contrast, a well-informed doctor will prescribe a combination of antibiotics for an ulcer patient to kill the bacteria that are now thought to cause most stomach ulcers.

The change in medical practice is due to general adoption in the 1990s of the theory that most peptic (gastric and duodenal) ulcers are caused by *Helicobacter pylori*, a species of bacteria that was discovered only in the early 1980s. When Barry Marshall and Robin Warren suggested that these bacteria might be responsible for peptic ulcers, their proposal was widely viewed as implausible, particularly by the specialists in gastroenterology who usually treat ulcers. But by the mid-1990s, medical consensus panels in many countries had endorsed the bacterial theory of peptic ulcers and their treatment by antibiotics.

How did this change take place? Contrast the following two pictures of scientific development. In a traditional view held by many scientists and philosophers, scientists conduct careful experiments and use the resulting observations to confirm or refute explanatory hypotheses that can provide objective knowledge about the world. In a postmodern view held by some sociologists and culture theorists, scientists conduct experiments to support the hypotheses that best suit their personal and social interests, and they negotiate with other scientists to accumulate sufficient power to ensure that their theories prevail over those of their rivals. Whereas on the traditional view science is largely a matter of logic, in the postmodern view it is largely a matter of politics. The traditional view is exemplified by such philosophers as Hempel (1965), Popper (1959), and Howson and Urbach (1989), whereas the postmodern view is found among sociologists and cultural theorists (e.g., Aronowitz 1988; Latour 1987; Ross 1996).

Neither the traditional nor the postmodern account provides much of an explanation of the discovery and acceptance of the bacterial theory of ulcers. The logical view neglects the diverse psychological and social processes that contribute to scientific development, whereas the political view ignores the extent to which the growth of science is affected by experimental interactions with the world and by rational assessment of alternative hypotheses. By discussing the ulcers case and other important events in the history of science and medicine, this book develops a much richer view of science as an integrated psychological, social, and physical system.

Many philosophers, historians, psychologists, and sociologists of science are concerned about explaining the development of scientific knowledge, but the kinds of explanations they propose are very diverse. Some philosophers of science prefer *logical* explanations, in which new scientific knowledge derives logically (inductively or deductively) from previous knowledge. Researchers in cognitive science, including psychologists, computer scientists, and some philosophers, propose *cognitive* explanations, in which the growth of knowledge derives from the mental structures and procedures of scientists. Sociologists of science offer *social* explanations, in which factors such as the organization and social interests of scientists are used to explain scientific change.

Are these explanations competitive or complementary? During the 1980s and 1990s, since sociologists of knowledge staked claims to what had been the traditional philosophical territory of explaining the growth of scientific knowledge, there has been conflict between proponents of logical and social explanations (see, for example, Barnes 1985; Bloor 1991; Brown 1984, 1989; Collins 1985). In the meantime, cognitive approaches have emerged with explanatory resources much richer than those available within the logical tradition, but the relation between cognitive and social accounts is rarely specified. Some sociologists are intensely antagonistic toward psychological and computational explanations, even going so far as to propose a ten-year moratorium on cognitive explanations of science (Latour and Woolgar 1986, p. 280). In a similar vein, Downes (1993) attacks what he calls "cognitive individualism" and defends the claim that scientific knowledge is socially produced.

But we can appreciate science as a product of individual minds *and* as a product of complex social organizations. Not only can we see cognitive and social explanations as providing complementary accounts of different aspects of science, but we can also look for ways of integrating those explanations, bringing them together in a common approach. This chapter compares cognitive and social explanation schemas and shows how they can be brought together to form integrated explanations of scientific change. To illustrate the unification of approaches, I show how a cognitive account of the chemical revolution can be socially enriched, and how a social account of the early development of science and mathematics can be cognitively enriched. The social categories of Downes (1993) require similar enrichment. Finally, I sketch how a cognitive/social approach offers new perspectives on the question of scientific rationality.

EXPLANATION SCHEMAS

An explanation schema consists of an explanation target, which is a question to be answered, and an explanatory pattern, which provides a general way of answering the question. For example, when you want to explain why a person is doing an action such as working long hours, you may employ the following rough explanation schema:

Action Explanation Schema

> *Explanation target:*
>> Why does a **person** with a set of **beliefs** and **desires** perform a particular **action**?
>
> *Explanatory pattern:*
>> The **person** has the **belief** that the **action** will help fulfill the **desires.**
>> This **belief** causes the **person** to pursue the **action**.

To apply this schema to a particular case, we replace the terms in boldface with specific examples, as in explaining Mary's action of working long hours in terms of her belief that this will help her to fulfill her desire to finish her PhD thesis. Many writers in the philosophy of science and cognitive science have described explanations and theories in terms of schemas, patterns, or other abstractions (Darden and Cain 1989; Giere 1994; Kelley 1972; Kitcher 1981, 1989, 1993; Leake 1992; Schaffner 1993; Schank 1986; Thagard 1988, 1992b).

What are the explanation targets in science studies? The most straightforward is belief change, as when we ask why eighteenth-century chemists adopted Antoine Lavoisier's oxygen theory or why nineteenth-century physicians adopted the germ theory of disease. The focus of the general explanation target is why scientists abandoned their previously held belief in favor of a new theory. But there is much more to the development of science than belief change, for we can ask why conceptual changes took place involving the introduction and reorganization of whole conceptual systems (see chapter 10).

Another legitimate explanation target in science studies involves discovery. Why did Lavoisier discover the oxygen theory in the 1770s? Why did Louis Pasteur discover the germ theory of disease in the 1860s? Although such questions are not open to logical explanations, they are grist for the mills of cognitive and social theorists (see chapter 3). Similarly, cognitive and social explanations can be given for why scientists pursue particular scientific research programs. Pursuit is an intermediate stage between the initial discovery or proposal of concepts and beliefs and their eventual acceptance. Within that stage, there are many interesting questions to be answered, such as why scientists conducted particular experiments in particular ways. The remainder of this chapter focuses on schemas for explaining belief change. But we should not forget that understanding science requires attention to other important explanation targets, such as conceptual change, discovery, and pursuit.

EXPLAINING BELIEF CHANGE

Why do scientists acquire new beliefs, sometimes abandoning old ones? My goal in this section is not to answer this question but rather to characterize the kinds of answers it has been given by means of logical, cognitive, and social explanation schemas. For all these schemas, the explanation target is as follows:

Why did a group of **scientists** adopt a particular set of **beliefs**?

But very different kinds of explanatory patterns can be used to answer this question.

For philosophers and others operating within the tradition of Frege and Russell, formal logic provides the central model for understanding knowledge, in a way roughly captured by the following schema.

Logical Explanation Schema

Explanation target:

Why did a group of **scientists** adopt a particular set of **beliefs**?

Explanatory pattern:

The **scientists** had a set of **previous beliefs**.

The **scientists** employed a **logical method**.

When applied to the **previous beliefs**, the **logical method** implies a set of **acquired beliefs**.

The **scientists** therefore adopted the **acquired beliefs**.

This schema can be made more specific by filling in the account of logical method, which might include deduction, confirmation theory, or—the currently most sophisticated candidate—Bayesian probability theory. Recent proponents of logical approaches to scientific change include Gärdenfors (1988), Howson and Urbach (1989), and Levi (1991). The logical positivists who originated this approach to understanding science were not so much concerned with explaining the growth of scientific knowledge as with providing a foundation for knowledge, but logical schemas have more recently been aimed at understanding scientific change.

Cognitive science offers a mentalistic explanatory approach that differs strongly from the antipsychologistic tradition of the logical positivists. It postulates that the human mind contains representational structures and computational processes that operate on these structures to produce new structures (Thagard 1996). These new structures include sentence-like beliefs as well as visual images and various kinds of concepts and schemas. Oversimplifying again, we can roughly capture cognitive explanations of belief change in a group of scientists as follows:

Cognitive Explanation Schema

  Explanation target:

    Why did a group of **scientists** adopt a particular set of **beliefs**?

  Explanatory pattern:

    The **scientists** had a set of **mental representations** that included a set of **previous beliefs**.

    The **scientists'** cognitive mechanisms included a set of **mental procedures**.

    When applied to the **mental representations** and **previous beliefs**, the **procedures** produce a set of **acquired beliefs**.

    So the **scientists** adopted the **acquired beliefs**.

This cognitive schema is more general than the logical one, since the representations and procedures that it invokes need not be those found in formal logic. Nonsentential representations such as diagrams, maps, and other visual images may be included among the scientists' mental representations in addition to sentential beliefs. Mental procedures may differ completely from methods in deductive and inductive logic and probability theory. For example, in my theory of explanatory coherence, beliefs are accepted on the basis of their coherence with other beliefs, and coherence is modeled computationally by means of connectionist algorithms that perform parallel satisfaction of multiple constraints (Thagard 1992b; see also chapter 4). The cognitive schema thus has a constraint that the antipsychologistic logical schema lacks: that the representations and procedures postulated must be plausible parts of human psychology. This constraint rules out both computationally intractable logical methods such as deductive closure and psychologically implausible methods such as Bayesian updating. Different cognitive explanations of scientific development have been offered by Churchland (1989), Darden (1991), Giere (1988), and Langley et al. (1987); for a collection of relevant papers, see Giere (1992).

Unlike logical methods, mental procedures can also explain the discovery of new concepts and hypotheses and decisions about the pursuit of research programs. Mental procedures can include those that we would not want to count as rational, such as motivated inference in which conclusions are affected by thinkers' personal goals (Kunda 1990). Thus, the cognitive schema competes with the logical schema for providing an understanding of science, since the procedures it postulates are by and large very different from logical methods. In principle, however cognitive and logical schemas could be compatible, if human belief change were fundamentally driven by logical mechanisms, but there is abundant evidence that human psychology involves a much broader range of structures and processes than logic describes (for deduction, see Johnson-Laird and Byrne 1991; for induction, see Holland et al. 1986).

Sociologists of science tend to focus on different features of science than on logical methods and mental procedures. They note that because of their social situations scientists have various interests, ranging from personal ambition to national sentiment. The also note that the development of science depends in part on the social connections that control information flow among scientists and the power relations that make some scientists much more influential than others in determining what science is done. Amalgamating ideas from various sociologists, we can roughly summarize various social explanations for belief change with the following:

Social Explanation Schema

    Explanation target:

        Why did a group of **scientists** adopt a particular set of **beliefs**?

    Explanatory pattern:

        The **scientists** had **previous beliefs** and **interests**.

        The **scientists** had **social connections** and **power relations**.

        Previous beliefs and **interests** and **social connections** and **power relations** lead to **acquired beliefs**.

        The **scientists** adopted the **acquired beliefs**.

This schema is incompatible with the logical schema, which assumes that epistemic matters must be kept isolated from psychological and sociological ones. However, it competes with the cognitive schema only if one assumes that the best explanation of the development of science must be either purely cognitive or purely social. But open-minded cognitivists can easily grant that scientists have the interests, social connections, and power relations postulated by sociologists, and that these qualities play some role in the development of science. Similarly, open-minded sociologists can grant that psychological structures and processes can mediate socially affected belief changes. The cognitive schema is incomplete because it fails to note how social relations can affect the spread of beliefs through the group of scientists. The social schema is incomplete because it fails to show how individual scientists came to acquire their beliefs.

A full account of the growth of scientific knowledge must therefore integrate the features of cognitive and social schemas, as is roughly illustrated by the following schema:

Integrated Cognitive-Social Explanation Schema

    Explanation target:

        Why did a group of **scientists** adopt a particular set of **beliefs**?

Explanatory pattern:

> The **scientists** had a set of **mental representations** that included a set of **previous beliefs** and a set of **interests**.
>
> The **scientists'** cognitive mechanisms included a set of **mental procedures**.
>
> The **scientists** had **social connections** and **power relations**.
>
> When applied to the **mental representations** and **previous beliefs** in the context of **social connections** and **power relations,** the **procedures** produce a set of **acquired beliefs**.
>
> The **scientists** adopted the **acquired beliefs**.

As with the previous schemas I presented, considerable detail must be added to put this explanation schema to work. To fill in the cognitive side, we must specify the mental representations and procedures that operate on them, including logical methods. To fill in the social side, we must specify the relevant social interests, connections, and power relations. As chapter 5 shows, it is also crucial to take into account the instruments and experiments through which scientists interact with the physical world.

To make the integrated cognitive-social explanation succeed, we must provide a much fuller account of how the cognitive and social features of scientists together determine their belief changes. For example, sociological explanations that appeal to the interests of scientists should be able to draw on Kunda's account (1990) of the cognitive mechanisms by which goals affect the selection of evidence. Her experiments show that, in general, people do not simply believe what they want to believe, but rather, that what they want to believe can influence their recall and use of evidence in more subtle ways that influence but do not fully determine their conclusions.

The question of how to make such integrated explanations work cannot be pursued abstractly, since the balance of cognitive and social factors is different in different historical cases. If the explanation target is why T. H. Huxley accepted Charles Darwin's theory of evolution by natural selection, cognitive factors such as the explanatory coherence of the theory should predominate, although the social relations of the two friends should not be ignored. On the other hand, if the explanation target is why some nineteenth-century U.S. industrialists embraced Social Darwinism, social factors such as the mesh between their economic interests and the idea of survival of the fittest should predominate, although the cognitive mechanisms of motivated inference must not be ignored. Similarly, the explanation for acceptance of hormonal or sociobiological explanations of behavioral sex differences may have to weight social values more heavily than evidence evaluation (Longino 1990). I now look in more detail at two important cases of the development of scientific knowledge: the chemical revolution and the development of the mathematical-mechanistic world view. These cases illustrate the interactions of cognitive and social factors whose contribution to medical knowledge are discussed at greater length in later chapters.

LAVOISIER AND THE CHEMICAL REVOLUTION

In previous work, I offered a cognitive account of the chemical revolution in which Lavoisier's oxygen theory of combustion overthrew the phlogiston theory of Georg Stahl (Thagard 1992b). This account has two parts; a description of the conceptual changes that took place when Lavoisier developed an alternative to the phlogiston scheme, and an explanation, in terms of explanatory coherence, of why he viewed the oxygen theory as superior to the phlogiston theory. Both parts are cognitive, in that conceptual schemes are taken to be organized systems of mental representations, and judgments of explanatory coherence are specified as psychologically plausible computational procedures. My account of the chemical revolution thus instantiates the cognitive schema presented earlier.

I remarked, however, that my account omitted the social side of the chemical revolution and did not presume to tell the whole story (Thagard 1992b, p. 113). What would a social explanation of the chemical revolution look like? My aim in what follows is not to provide a full social account of the acceptance of the oxygen theory but merely to sketch enough that the compatibility and integrability of social and cognitive explanations become evident. From a social perspective, we can look at the developments of Lavoisier's own beliefs and also at how these beliefs spread to the larger scientific community. Social treatments of the chemical revolution include those of Levin (1984), McCann (1978), and Perrin (1987, 1988); other useful sources include Conant (1964), Donovan (1988), Guerlac (1961), and Holmes (1985).

No scientist is an island. Lavoisier had numerous teachers, friends, and associates who contributed to the development of his ideas. We can mention, for example, Guyton de Morveau, who demonstrated to Lavoisier in 1772 that metals gain weight when calcined; Joseph Priestley, who showed Lavoisier in 1774 his experiments that mercury when heated forms a red "calx"; and his wife, Marie, who translated English articles for him, made entries in his notebooks, and drew figures for his publications. Lavoisier was elected at a young age (25 years) to the French Academy and participated in its meetings. He also had a smaller circle of chemists with whom he could perform experiments and discuss the defects of the phlogiston theory uninhibitedly at a time when senior chemists such as Philippe Macquer would not have approved of the aggressive proposal of an alternative theory. Although he alone wrote his most important publications on the oxygen theory, he had various other joint publications, including the influential *Method of Chemical Nomenclature* (1787), written with Guyton de Morveau, Berthollet, and Fourcroy.

Lavoisier's broader social situation also contributed to his work. His substantial income as a tax farmer meant that he had ample resources and time to conduct his experiments (although this position ultimately led to his execution during the French Revolution). According to an early biographer, "His great wealth, his excellent education, his mathematical precision, his general views, and his persevering industry, all contributed to ensure his success" (Thomson 1813, p. 82). Understanding how the spread of oxygen theory differed between France and England requires an appreciation of the institutional differences between the two countries, which McEvoy summarizes:

> The difference between Lavoisier's corporate view of knowledge and Priestley's individualistic epistemology highlights the difference between the institutional organization of French and British science in the late eighteenth century. In the highly organized and centralized community of France, the pressures of formal education, centralized learned societies, employment opportunities, and a competitive system of reward and recognition meant that aspiring French chemists had little choice but to follow the intellectual lead of the academicians in Paris. In contrast, the organization of English science was much weaker, comprising fewer educational institutions, decentralized societies, little employment opportunity, and a looser congregation of amateurs with closer ties to entrepreneurial industry than their French contemporaries. Thus, whereas the highly integrated community of state-subsidized French theoreticians provided fertile ground for the flowering of paradigmatic conformity during the Chemical Revolution, the dissemination of Lavoisier's theory in England met with a more varied resistance. (McEvoy 1988, pp. 210–211)

Thus, a full explanation of the development of the oxygen theory should not be limited to conceptual development and belief revision, as in my cognitive account. Nevertheless, there is no incompatibility between that account and the relevant social information. No matter how much is said about how Lavoisier gained information from his associates or about how his social situation inclined him to act in certain ways, there remains the problem of describing how his conceptual system developed and changed as he formed and adopted the oxygen theory of combustion, rejecting the phlogiston theory that he had held as a young chemist. As is displayed in the Integrated Cognitive-Social Explanation Schema, cognitive and social explanations of conceptual change can coexist.

Both mind and society contributed to the development of the oxygen theory, but they do not tell the whole story either. The experiments of de Morveau, Lavoisier, Priestley, and others were an important part of the development of eighteenth-century chemistry: Neither mental nor social construction can fully explain why experiments on combustion and calcination gave the results they did. The growth of scientific knowledge is a function of mind, society, *and* the world. The difficult task for science studies is to create a synthetic account of how mind, society, and the world interactively contribute to scientific development.

The social side of the chemical revolution becomes even more prominent if one addresses the question of how scientists other than Lavoisier came to adopt the oxygen theory. Contrary to the common view that adoption of a revolutionary theory comes only when the proponents of the previous theory die off, the oxygen theory was almost universally adopted in France and (more slowly) in England by scientists who had to abandon their previous phlogiston beliefs. A cognitive explanation of this switch goes roughly like this. Through personal contact with Lavoisier or his disciples, or through reading his argumentative publications, scientists began mentally to acquire the new scientific conceptual scheme. The new mental representations enabled them to understand Lavoisier's claims and to appreciate that the oxygen theory has greater explanatory coherence than the phlogiston theory. This appreciation was part of a cognitive process that led them to accept the oxygen theory, abandoning the phlogiston theory and its conceptual scheme.

From a social perspective, we want to know more about how information spread from scientist to scientist. Diffusion of the oxygen theory was slow, even in France (Perrin 1988). Members of Lavoisier's immediate circle, such as Pierre Laplace, were fairly quick to adopt his views, but the majority of French chemists came around only in the late 1780s and early 1790s. According to Perrin, nearly all converts initially resisted Lavoisier's theory but underwent a conversion that lasted several years. The duration of conversion has both a cognitive and a social explanation. The cognitive explanation is that developing a new conceptual system and appreciating its superiority to the old one is a difficult mental operation; the social explanation is that information flow in social networks is far from instantaneous. Lavoisier and his fellow antiphlogistinians worked to improve the flow—by giving lectures and demonstrations, by publishing articles and books, and by starting a new journal, *Annales de Chimie*. It is also possible that different scientists had different interests that made them resistant to the new theories, although I know of no documentation of this. It is certainly true that different scientists had different initial beliefs and cognitive resources. My cognitive account of Lavoisier cannot be automatically transferred over to all the other scientists, since they had different starting points and associated beliefs. In principle, we would need a different cognitive account for each scientist; but these accounts would have a great deal in common, since the scientists shared many concepts and beliefs, not to mention similar underlying cognitive processes.

Thus, there is much more to a social account of the chemical revolution than was present in my cognitive explanation of Lavoisier. However, the expanded social account must coalesce with cognitive descriptions of Lavoisier and all the other scientists whose beliefs and conceptual systems changed.

HADDEN ON THE MATHEMATICAL-MECHANISTIC WORLD VIEW

Despite the antagonism that some sociologists display toward psychology, many sociological explanations of scientific developments can be usefully supplemented by cognitive explanations. As an illustration, consider the socio-logical account of some essential features of early modern mechanistic thought given by Richard Hadden. His abstract provides a summary (Hadden 1988, p. 255): "A sociological explanation is offered for certain features of the mathematical-mechanistic world view. Relations of commodity production and exchange are seen as providing an analogy of 'abstraction' for such a world view. The mediation between social relations and content of science is provided by commercial reckoners who contributed a new meaning to ancient mathematical concepts and thus paved the way for the notion that all sensually intuitable events are explicable in terms of the motion of qualitatively similar bodies." The explanation target here is the emergence in the fifteenth and six-teenth centuries of the view that nature can be understood mechanically and mathematically.

Hadden argues that social relations involving commercial arithmetic pro-vided an analogy for how nature could be understood. "The crux of my argu-ment is that a view of the conditions of the period gets projected onto all of nature and eventually human society as well" (Hadden 1988, p. 257). Just as in the early modern European economy the sensible properties of commodities such as bread and shoes could be abstracted into exchange values, so the sensi-ble properties of all physical objects could be ignored in favor of their mechan-ical and mathematical properties. Hadden provides evidence that such de-velopments as the replacement of ancient concepts of number were influenced by commercial concerns. Simon Stevin, for example, who was among the first to introduce the notion of decimal fractions, was very much concerned with practical mathematical problems.

Without evaluating the plausibility of Hadden's Marxian account, we can readily see that it presupposes cognitive processes. His explanation of the emergence of new mathematical ideas assumes that "social relations provided analogies and metaphors which were refined technically by thinkers whose concerns involved, at first, the reckoning up of calculable aspects of those relations" (Hadden 1988, p. 271). Thinkers such as Stevin, Hadden conjec-tures, used commercial social relations as analogs to develop ideas about mathematics and science. Although Hadden's documentation of Stevin's use of analogy is sparse, later uses of social analogies in science have been well established. Darwin, for example, came up with the idea for natural selection by reading Malthus on political economy (Darwin 1958). It has also been conjectured that Lavoisier's innovative concern with conservation of matter may have been influenced by his tax farmer's familiarity with the balance sheet.

Although Hadden says nothing about how analogical thinking actually works, this is where cognitive science has much to offer, since the topic has been thoroughly investigated using psychological experiments and computational models. The process most relevant to Hadden's account is *analogical mapping*, in which some of the content of a source analog is transferred to a target analog. In Hadden's case study, the target analog involves the mathematics and physics of objects, and the antecedently understood source analog involves commercial and social objects. According to Holyoak and Thagard's theory of mapping (1989, 1995), people's cognitive processes in mapping from one domain to the other require simultaneous satisfaction of semantic, structural, and pragmatic constraints. Some kind of cognitive theory is presupposed by sociological explanations such as Hadden's, which see analogy as the mediating factor between social relations and the development of science. Cognitive theories of analogy are not alternatives to Hadden's account—the social and economic relations he discusses are an important, ineliminable part of the story. But cognitive explanations supplement the social ones by describing the mental processes of the thinkers who made the transition to new ideas. For more on analogy, see chapter 9.

Latour and Woolgar (1986) pursue their extreme anticognitive stance by ignoring the content of scientific papers and speaking only of how scientists use "inscriptions" to produce other inscriptions, as if all that mattered to the process of scientific development were the social relations of scientists and the papers they shuffle around. Latour and Woolgar clearly miss an important part of what is going on when the cognitive representations and processes of scientists enable them to read what has been written, develop and test new hypotheses, and produce new writings. A sociologist or historian who ponders scientific development without paying attention to the intellectual goals and cognitive processes of the scientists involved is like an anthropologist who does fieldwork in an alien tribe without knowing the language. Like Hadden, Latour and Woolgar can only gain from cognitive models that provide a crucial supplement to their social accounts of what laboratory scientists are doing. As Bloor pointed out in the second edition of one of the books that spawned the sociology of scientific knowledge (1991, p. 168), sociologists would be "foolish" to deny the need for a background theory about individual cognitive processes. Similarly, Barnes et al. (1996) present a sociological approach to science that is also open to philosophical and psychological approaches.

ALTERNATIVES TO COGNITIVE INDIVIDUALISM

Downes (1993, p. 452) accuses me and others of *cognitive individualism*, "the thesis that a sufficient explanation for all cognitive activity will be provided by an account of autonomous individual cognitive agents." Obviously, I do not hold this position and in fact have given a battery of arguments for why psychological reductionism in science studies is bound to fail (see chapter 14). But the kind of anticognitive view that Downes seems to prefer in alliance with Latour, Woolgar, and Collins is also bound to fail. Downes distinguishes three levels of social aspects of science, each of which can be shown to have an essential cognitive component.

The first level is the "public embodiment of scientific theories," which includes the textbooks, research papers, instruments, and other shared property of the scientific community. These things clearly exist outside the mental representations of individual scientists, and naturalistic science studies cannot ignore their significance. But part of this significance is cognitive: The use of textbooks, papers and instruments by scientists presupposes scientists' mental capacities to read, write, plan, design, and in other ways produce and use such tools. The public embodiment of scientific knowledge would be pointless if scientists lacked the cognitive processes to understand and produce the embodied objects. Use of external representations such as books and diagrams means that the thought of each scientist does not have to rely entirely on his or her own internal mental representations; but internal representations are needed to comprehend the external ones.

Downes's second level is social interaction, such as is found in complex laboratory work in which no one researcher is entirely responsible for the ultimate result. This level is indeed of great importance, as is clear from research in fields such as psychology, in which most research is collaborative, and experimental physics, in which almost all work is collaborative. But the importance of collaboration and social interaction speaks only against the most implausible forms of psychological reductionism and provides no support for purely social accounts (see chapter 11). Understanding how scientists work with each other in part requires understanding how they communicate with each other, which in turn requires cognitive theories of how they represent information and use language and other means, such as diagrams to convey information to each other. Level 2 is undeniably social, but it is also undeniably cognitive.

Downes's third social level depends on the claim that the activities of scientists make sense only when taken in the context of a broader scientific community. The difference between someone performing an experiment and someone else doing the same physical motions in a play lies in the fact that the former is part of a community of experimenters. We can grant this social distinction,

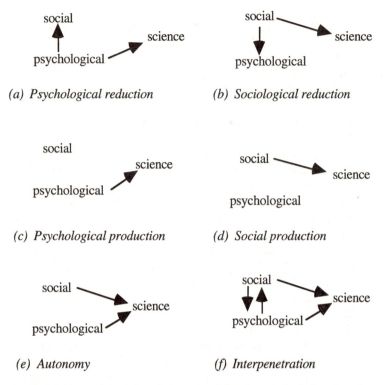

Figure 1.1. Six models of the relation of social and psychological explanations of science. The arrows signify "explains."

but we cannot help but notice that there are also obvious cognitive distinctions. The mental representations of the trained scientist are drastically different from those of the actor who is merely mouthing lines, since the scientists have absorbed an enormous amount of both declarative and procedural knowledge in the course of training. The ability of the experimenter to plan experiments and interpret the results cannot be explained purely in terms of social context but must also make reference to mental structures and procedures.

My arguments that Downes's three social levels each have a crucial cognitive aspect are in no way an attempt to explain them psychologically. We can appreciate social aspects of science at each of these levels while simultaneously appreciating relevant cognitive aspects. Figure 1.1 illustrates six possible relations between psychological and social explanations of science. Schemas *a* and *b* express extreme views about the dominance of a particular style of explanation. Psychological reductionism (*a*) is the view that everything about science, including social aspects, can be understood in terms of the psychology of the individuals involved. An analog of this view may survive in the economic doctrine of methodological individualism, which proclaims the reduction of macroeconomics to microeconomics, but I know of no one in science studies who holds this view. Sociological reductionism (*b*) is the view that everything about science, including its psychological aspects, can be understood in terms of social factors. In their most rhetorical moments, some Marxists and social constructivists approximate to this view. A slightly more modest view (*d*) advocates social explanations of science but does not purport to explain the psychological. Similarly, schema *c* proposes to simply ignore the social explanations while providing psychological explanations of science. The last two schemas (*e* and *f*) present less dogmatic views of the relation of mind and society. Schema *e* eclectically proposes that social and psychological explanations of science can proceed in relative autonomy of science, perhaps explaining different aspects of science, whereas schema *f* presents a potentially richer and more dynamic view of science studies, in which the social and the psychological are mutually informed. The task before us is to specify these interactions in much more detail, as chapters 3 to 6 do for the development and acceptance of the bacterial theory of ulcers.

The best strategy for naturalistic studies of science is neither psychological reductionism nor sociological reductionism but an integrated approach that takes both the cognitive and the social seriously. To conclude this chapter, I argue that such an approach can be normative—prescritive of how science should be done—as well as descriptive of how it is done.

MIND, SOCIETY, AND RATIONALITY

When the sociology of scientific knowledge arose in the 1970s with its implication of supplanting logical explanation schemas with social ones, philosophers were aghast. Philosophers in the analytic tradition have viewed incursions of psychology into epistemology as assaults on rationality. Incursions of sociology seemed even worse, especially given the rampant relativism of sociologists such as Woolgar (1988), who think that scientific objectivity is an illusion. However, as epistemology and philosophy of science have come to take psychology more seriously, it has become obvious that psychologism requires new theories of rationality but need not embrace irrationalism or relativism. For example, Giere (1988), Goldman (1986), Harman (1986), and Thagard (1988, 1992b) all use psychology to challenge traditional logic-based conceptions of rationality while opening up new territory for rational appraisal.

Similarly, taking the social context of science seriously does not entail relativism. Goldman (1992, p. 194), Kitcher (1993), and Solomon (1994) have outlined how social practices, like cognitive processes, can be subject to rational appraisal, for example, concerning the extent to which they promote reliable beliefs. Logical explanation schemas carry rationality with them for free, since any beliefs that are inferred logically are presumably warranted. With cognitive and social explanations, the matter is more complicated. We have to ask first what is the best cognitive and social account of a scientific development and only then raise the question of whether the cognitive and social processes invoked are ones that promote the ends of science. In pursuit of the first question, philosophers of science can ally themselves with psychologists, sociologists, and historians of science who, lacking an appetite for the second question, may choose to leave concern for rationality in philosophy, its traditional home. But rational appraisal of social practices and organizations has barely begun (see Goldman 1992, and chapters 11 to 13 of this text).

Solomon (1994) has made the audacious proposal that the scientific community, rather than the individual scientist, should be taken as the important unit of cognitive processing. She contends that a scientific community may reach a consensus that can be judged to be normatively correct from an empirical perspective, even though not one individual scientist in the community made an unbiased judgment. Although the view that she calls "social empiricism" is a useful antidote to past neglect of social aspects of rationality, it swings too far in that direction. My Integrated Cognitive-Social Explanation Schema allows various cognitive and motivational biases to influence the judgments of scientists. But if these biases are as dominant as Solomon suggests, it becomes mysterious how the community collectively reaches a consensus based on empirical success rather than on communal delusion. On the other hand, if scientists share cognitive processes such as those postulated by my theory of explanatory coherence (Thagard 1992b), then their convergence on the empirically successful theory despite their disparate individual biases becomes intelligible. Individual evaluations of the merits of competing theories are not all there is to rationality, but they are an indispensable part of it.

A key conclusion to draw from the interdependence of cognitive and social explanations of scientific change is that the appraisal of cognitive and social strategies must also be linked. Cognitive appraisal should consider the fact that much scientific knowledge is collaborative, and we should therefore evaluate particular cognitive strategies in part on the basis of how well they promote collaboration (see chapter 11). Conversely, social appraisal should take into account the cognitive capacities and limitations of the individuals whose interaction produces knowledge. Determining how to facilitate the growth of scientific knowledge, like the more descriptive task of explaining this development, depends on appreciating the complex interdependencies of mind and society. The next five chapters, however, are primarily descriptive and attempt to explain the development and acceptance of the bacterial theory of ulcers. I return to the question of social rationality in chapters 11 to 14.

SUMMARY

Philosophers, psychologists, and sociologists have offered alternative explanations of the development of scientific knowledge. Cognitive and social explanations can, however, be complementary rather than competitive, and can be combined to fit an Integrated Cognitive-Social Explanation Schema that incorporates both mental processes and social relations. Cognitive accounts of scientific change need to be supplemented with social explanations, just as social accounts need to be supplemented with cognitive explanations. Like cognitive processes, social processes can be evaluated according to how well they contribute to the growth of knowledge.

CHAPTER 2

Explaining Disease

TWO KINDS of explanation are important in medicine. When a patient goes to a physician with a set of complaints and symptoms, the physician's first task is to make a diagnosis of a disease that explains the symptoms. For example, if the patient has a fever, muscle aches, and a runny nose, the physician may explain these symptoms by saying that the patient has influenza. The second kind of explanation, which belongs to medical research rather than clinical practice, requires an answer to the question of why the patient became sick with influenza, which we now know is caused by a virus. Over the past one hundred and fifty years, medical science has identified and generated explanations for numerous human diseases.

This chapter shows that the explanations furnished by medical research fall under a set of basic patterns or schemas that specify the causes of various kinds of disease. After describing the humoral theory that was central to medicine up to the middle of the nineteenth century, I outline the germ theory of disease as a system of explanation schemas. Nutritional and autoimmune diseases are characterized by patterns of explanation that specify nongerm causes for diseases. During the 1980s and 1990s, advances in molecular genetics have generated new explanation patterns for diseases such as cancer. Theoretical knowledge in medicine is not like physics, in which a small number of mathematical equations can provide unified explanations of many observed phenomena. Medicine provides unifications of a different kind, by means of an organized collection of explanation schemas that characterize the causes of numerous diseases.

EXPLANATION SCHEMAS IN THE HISTORY OF MEDICINE

At the most general level, a medical explanation schema has the following form:

Disease Explanation Schema

  Explanation target:

    Why does a **patient** have a **disease** with associated **symptoms**?

  Explanatory pattern:

    The **patient** is or has been subject to **causal factors**.

    The **causal factors** produce the **disease** and **symptoms**.

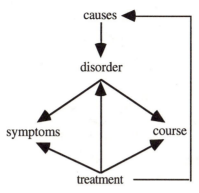

Figure 2.1. Causal structure of disease concepts. The arrows
in this and subsequent figures indicate causal relations.

In this schema, the terms in boldface are to be replaced with particular patients, diseases, and so on. At this level of generality, the disease explanation is not useful, but schemas for infectious, nutritional, and other kinds of diseases have provided powerful means of medical explanation.

Disease explanation schemas can alternatively be represented by diagrams that display the causal relations that characterize a disease, as shown by Figure 2.1. Symptoms are the observable manifestations of a disease, which can develop over time in particular ways that constitute the expected course of the disease. The symptoms arise from the cause or causes (etiology) of the disease. Treatment of the disease should affect the symptoms and course of the disease, often by affecting the causal factors that produce the symptoms. For example, tuberculosis has a set of typical symptoms such as coughing and the growth of tubercles (nodules) in the lungs and elsewhere, along with a course that before the twentieth century often included wasting and death. The disorder most commonly affects the lungs, but tuberculosis can also infect many other parts of the body. In 1882, Robert Koch discovered that the cause of tuberculosis is a bacterium, now called *Mycobacterium tuberculosis*, and in 1932, Gerhard Domagk discovered that this microbe can be killed by the drug Prontosil. The drug streptomycin was discovered in 1944 and proved effective in treating the disease. Hence, today tuberculosis has a well-understood cause and a kind of treatment that is effective except for the emergence of bacterial strains resistant to antibiotics.

Hippocrates and the Humoral Theory

The first scientific disease explanation schema is due to Hippocrates, who was born on the Greek island of Cos around 460 B.C. We know little concerning what he himself wrote, but between 430 and 330 B.C., he and his disciples

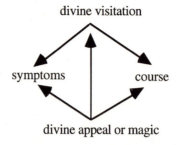

Figure 2.2. Causal structure of religious disease concepts.

produced a body of medical writing. The Hippocratic approach to medicine, as interpreted by Galen and others, dominated European medical thought well into the nineteenth century.

Hippocrates developed a naturalistic approach to medicine that contrasted sharply with the religious views that preceded him. Figure 2.2 shows the causal network that the Hippocratics rejected, for example, in their discussion of the "sacred disease," epilepsy. In the traditional view, epilepsy was caused by divine visitation and hence could only be cured by using an appeal to the gods or other magic. Little was said of the existence of a physical disorder responsible for the observable symptoms. The Hippocratics argued that epilepsy is no more sacred than any other disease and contended that it is caused by an excess of phlegm, one of the four humors (fluids) that constitute the human body.

The following quotes from Hippocratic treatises concisely summarize the humoral theory:

> The human body contains blood, phlegm, yellow bile, and black bile. These are the things that make up its constitution and cause its pains and health. Health is primarily that state in which these constituent substances are in the correct proportion to each other, both in strength and quantity, and are well mixed. (Lloyd 1978, p. 262)

> All human diseases arise from bile and phlegm; the bile and phlegm produce diseases when, inside the body, one of them becomes too moist, too dry, too hot, or too cold; they become this way from foods and drinks, from exertions and wounds, from smell, sound, sight, and venery, and from heat and cold. (Hippocrates 1988, p. 7)

To modern ears, the humoral theory sounds bizarre, but in its time it possessed considerable conceptual and explanatory coherence. Many of Hippocrates's contemporaries believed in four fundamental elements: earth, air, fire, and water. These elements possess various combinations of the four qualities of moist, dry, hot, and cold; for example, fire is hot and dry. The four humors also possess these qualities in different degrees, so that bile tends to be hot and phlegm tends to be cold.

According to the Hippocratics, diseases arise because of humoral imbalances. Too much bile, for example, can produce various fevers, and too much phlegm can cause epilepsy or angina. Imbalances arise from natural causes such as heredity (e.g., phlegmatic parents have phlegmatic children), regimen (e.g., diet and other behavior), and climate (e.g., temperature, wind, and moisture conditions). Different kinds of imbalance produce different diseases with symptoms and development that were acutely observed by the Hippocratics. The Hippocratics described in detail not only the symptoms of patients with a particular disease but also the ways that the patients tended to develop toward recovery or death. The course of a disease was affected by the development of a particular humor, producing crises that signaled basic changes in patient outcome. Fevers were classified as tertian, quartan, and so on based on the number of days before a crisis occurred.

Hippocratic treatment of a disease attempted to address either the causes of the humoral imbalance, by changing diet and environment, or the humoral balance itself. To rid the body of excess bile or phlegm, methods were used to induce vomiting or evacuation of the bowels, and veins were opened to let blood. The use of emetics, purgatives, and phlebotomy remained standard medical practice well into the nineteenth century. These techniques make sense within the Hippocratic framework because they are means of changing fluid balances. Figure 2.3 displays the structure of the causal network underlying the Hippocratic concept of disease.

The Hippocratic theory of disease causation translates into the following explanation schema:

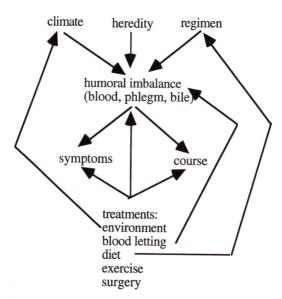

Figure 2.3. Causal structure of Hippocratic disease concepts.

Humoral Theory Explanation Schema

   Explanation target:

   Why does a **patient** have a **disease** with associated **symptoms**?

   Explanatory pattern:

     The body of the **patient** contains four humors: blood, phlegm, yellow bile, and black bile.

     Nutritional and environmental **factors** produce a **humoral imbalance**.

     The **humoral imbalance** produces the **disease** and **symptoms**.

In the Hippocratic view, different diseases arise from different humoral imbalances. For example, various fevers arise from too much bile, and epilepsy and angina are the result of too much phlegm. Thus, the humoral explanation schema can be instantiated for particular diseases, as in this explanation pattern for epilepsy:

Epilepsy Explanation Schema:

   Explanation target:

   Why does a **patient** have epilepsy characterized by seizures?

   Explanatory pattern:

     The body of the **patient** contains an excess of phlegm.

     The excess of phlegm in the **patient** produces the epileptic seizures.

This schema can in turn be instantiated to explain why a particular patient is sick. Thus, medical explanation in the humoral theory was provided by a hierarchy of schemas that applied general beliefs about disease causation to particular cases.

Pasteur and the Germ Theory

The major blow to the humoral theory came in the 1860s, when Louis Pasteur and others developed the germ theory of disease. Pasteur was a French chemist who in the 1850s turned his attention to the process of fermentation, including the production of lactic acid in sour milk and the production of alcohol in wine and beer. Many scientists at the time believed that fermentation and putrefaction were the result of spontaneous generation. Justus von Liebig, for example, contended in 1839 that fermentation in beer is not caused by yeast but by the internal development of the beer. Pasteur was able to show that the yeast increased in weight, nitrogen, and carbon content during fermentation, and he inferred that yeast is a living organism that is the cause of fermentation in beer and wine. Pasteur proceeded in the early 1860s to identify other organisms—bacteria—that produce lactic acid fermentation. To challenge directly the theory of spontaneous generation, he conducted ingenious experiments to show that fermentation does not take place in the absence of contamination by air. Pasteur's work greatly improved the manufacture of vinegar and wine, and he

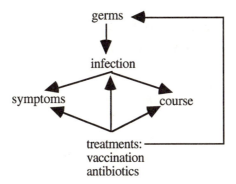

Figure 2.4. Causal structure of the germ theory of disease.

was invited in 1865 to investigate an epidemic of silkworm disease in the south of France. He also took time to study cholera, which had spread to France from Egypt. Naturally, Pasteur applied to silkworms some of the same microscopic techniques that had proved so fertile in his studies of fermentation.

Pasteur (and, independently, the British surgeon Joseph Lister) made the most important mental leap in the history of medicine, pursuing an analogy between fermentation and disease. They realized that just as fermentation is caused by yeast and bacteria, so diseases may also be caused by microorganisms. (See chapter 9 for a discussion of this and other analogies.) In the second half of the nineteenth century, bacteria were shown to be the cause of many important human diseases, including tuberculosis, cholera, and gonorrhea. The germ theory employed a concept of disease (figure 2.4) and an explanation schema that differed dramatically from that of the humoral theory:

Germ Theory Explanation Schema:

   Explanation target:
   Why does a **patient** have a **disease** with **symptoms** such as fever?
   Explanatory pattern:
   The **patient** has been infected by a **microbe.**
   The **microbe** produces the **disease** and **symptoms**.

Different kinds of microbes provide variants of the Germ Theory Explanation Schema, which was originally based on bacteria. By the 1890s, it was known that some disease-causing microbes were too small to be observed with the microscope; but what we now call viruses were observed in 1939 using electron microscopes (see chapter 10). Other infectious microbes include protozoa and fungi. In the 1980s, Prusiner hypothesized that spongiform encephalopathies such as scrapie, kuru, and Creutzfeldt-Jakob disease were caused by a novel kind of infectious agent called a *prion* (see chapter 8). We can describe current knowledge about infectious diseases in terms of the hierarchy of explanation schemas shown in Figure 2.5. Falling under the Germ Theory Explana-

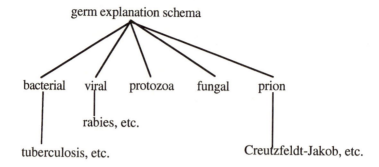

Figure 2.5. Hierarchy of infectious disease schemas.

tion Schema are at least five more specific schemas for bacterial, viral, and other kinds of infectious diseases. Particular diseases then fall under the schemas for different kinds of infectious microbes; for numerous examples, see Murray et al. (1994).

The germ theory of disease has been frequently mentioned since the 1860s, but it is difficult to state in terms of universal laws or general models. Instead, we can think of the germ theory in terms of the hierarchy of schemas (figure 2.5), which includes the general Germ Theory Explanation Schema, explanation schemas for classes of infectious diseases caused by different agents, and schemas for particular diseases. This collection of schemas provides an excellent, unifying fit with hundreds of human maladies.

Nutritional Diseases

Scientific advances in the first half of the twentieth century identified an entirely different class of noninfectious diseases caused by vitamin deficiencies (Funk 1912; see chapter 8). In 1928, for example, Albert Szent-Györgyi isolated vitamin C, deprivation of which causes bleeding gums and other symptoms of scurvy. The explanation schema for nutritional diseases is as follows:

Nutritional Disease Explanation Schema:
  Explanation target:
    Why does a **patient** have a **disease** with associated **symptoms**?
  Explanatory pattern:
    The **patient** has a deficiency of a needed **nutrient.**
    Absence of the **nutrient** produced the **disease** and the **symptoms.**

In addition to being applicable to scurvy and vitamin C (see chapter 8), this schema fits such diseases as beriberi, which is due to vitamin B_1 deficiency, and rickets, which is due to vitamin D deficiency. As with infectious diseases, the clinical importance of explanation schemas is that they suggest therapies, such as treating scurvy with vitamin C supplements and treating bacterial infections with antibiotics.

Autoimmune Diseases

During the 1950s, medical researchers led by Frank Macfarlane Burnet developed an understanding of how the body's immune system helps protect it against infectious agents (Silverstein 1989). This understanding generated a new class of diseases that occur when the immune system becomes overactive and attacks the body it is supposed to protect. For example, Grave's disease appears to originate when the immune system damages the thyroid, and lupus erythematosus is the result of an immune attack on the connective tissue. Other diseases that may have autoimmune origins include multiple sclerosis (in which there is damage to myelin in the central nervous system), rheumatic fever (in which there is damage to joint cartilage), and juvenile diabetes (in which there is damage to the pancreas) (Wyngaarden et al. 1992). Here is the general explanation pattern:

Autoimmune Disease Explanation Schema:
  Explanation target:
    Why does a **patient** have a **disease** with associated **symptoms**?
  Explanatory pattern:
    The **patient's immune system** attacks an infectious agent.
    The **immune system** becomes overactive and attacks **bodily tissues**.
    Damage to the **bodily tissues** produces the **symptoms**.

Advances in the understanding of infectious, nutritional, and autoimmune diseases have been monumental, but they leave many of the most important medical problems unexplained. Atherosclerosis, cancer, adult-onset diabetes, and osteoarthritis are just some of the widespread diseases whose primary causes do not appear to be infectious agents, nutritional deficiencies, or autoimmune reactions.

EXPLANATION SCHEMAS FROM MOLECULAR GENETICS

During the 1980s and 1990s, the explanation of disease has undergone major transformations owing to developments in molecular genetics. According to Edward Rubenstein (1994, p. vii):

> We are in the midst of revolutionary changes in basic science that will allow us to identify and to correct or circumvent molecular defects that give rise to some of

the most prevalent afflictions of humanity, including many forms of atherosclerosis, hypertension, diabetes, neoplasia, autoimmune diseases, and disorders of mendelian inheritance. Henceforth, clinicians will increasingly employ diagnostic methods and therapeutic interventions made possible by the manipulation of the genes of microorganisms, plants, animals, and humans. In short, we have entered the era of molecular medicine.

Medical explanations based on molecular genetics are very different from the kinds of germ-based and nutrition-based explanations of diseases that became available after the mid-nineteenth century.

Molecular genetics has a general explanation schema with specialized versions that apply to diseases of various kinds, including those caused by defects in single genes, multifactorial diseases, and cancer. The following schema is abstracted from Strachan and Read (1996):

Molecular Genetics Disease Explanation Schema:
   Explanation target:
      Why does a **patient** get a **disease** with associated **symptoms**?
   Explanatory pattern:
      Genes in the **patient**'s body are encoded in **DNA**.
      DNA specifies the synthesis of **RNA**.
      RNA specifies the synthesis of polypeptides, which form **proteins**.
      Normal function of a **patient**'s body requires the production of **proteins**.
      Mutations produce changes in **DNA**.
      Mutated **DNA** may alter the production of **proteins** needed for normal functioning of the **patient**'s body.
      Abnormal functioning in the **patient** produces the **disease** and its **symptoms**.

This schema leaves open whether mutations are inherited or, as in most cancers, occur during a patient's lifetime. It also leaves open whether the alteration of protein production involves a loss of function, as in most inherited diseases, or a gain of function found in cancer growth. This style of explanation, obviously very different from the infectious and other disease explanations presented in the last section, is too general to apply to particular diseases, which fall into several different classes. The diseases most easily understood in terms of molecular genetics are those produced by defects in single genes.

Mendelian Diseases

A *Mendelian* genetic character is one whose presence or absence depends on the genotype (types of alleles) at a single chromosomal locus. In humans, more than five thousand Mendelian characters have been identified, including hundreds of inherited diseases (McKusick and Francomano 1994). A Mendelian disease is one caused by an inherited mutation in a single gene, yielding the following kind of explanation schema:

Mendelian Disease Explanation Schema

> *Explanation target:*
> Why does a **patient** get a **disease** with associated **symptoms**?
> *Explanatory pattern:*
> The **patient** has inherited a mutated **gene**.
> The mutated **gene** is defective and produces the **disease** and its **symptoms**.

This schema is a specialization of the more abstract Molecular Genetics Disease Explanation Schema, in that it states that a single inherited gene is responsible for the disease. The first disease to be identified as genetic in origin, in 1902, was alkaptonuria, a rare disorder characterized by large quantities of dark-colored urine.

Further specifications of the Mendelian Disease Explanation Schema are possible because of the five different patterns of Mendelian inheritance: autosomal dominant, autosomal recessive, X-linked dominant, X-linked recessive, and Y-linked. The following schema, specifies an autosonal recessive disease:

Autosomal Recessive Disease Explanation Schema

> *Explanation target:*
> Why does a **patient** get a **disease** with associated **symptoms**?
> *Explanatory pattern:*
> The **patient** has inherited a recessive mutated **gene** from both parents.
> The mutated **gene** is defective and produces the **disease** and its **symptoms**.

This schema is now specific enough that it applies to particular diseases such as cystic fibrosis:

Cystic Fibrosis Explanation Schema

> *Explanation target:*
> Why does a patient get **cystic fibrosis** with **symptoms** such as excessive mucous and pulmonary failure?
> *Explanatory pattern:*
> The patient has inherited a mutated gene ΔF508 from both parents.
> The mutated gene ΔF508 produces anomalous mucous **secretions**.
> These **secretions** produce **symptoms** such as excessive mucous and pulmonary failure.

At this level, it is now possible to explain, in a manner that is virtually deductive, why a particular patient became sick: With few exceptions, every human

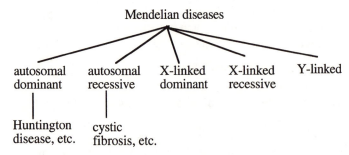

Figure 2.6. Hierarchy of Mendelian disease schemas.

who has inherited the mutated gene ΔF508 from both parents eventually gets cystic fibrosis. Medical explanations are rarely so simple, however, as the discussion of more complex diseases will show. The human genome contains about seventy thousand genes, but only about five thousand Mendelian phenotypes are known (Strachan and Read 1996). Most diseases involve the action of more than one gene, and some genes are responsible for more than one disease. For example, the gene PRNP is implicated in both Creutzfeldt-Jakob syndrome and familial fatal insomnia. The schemas for Mendelian diseases form the hierarchy shown in Figure 2.6.

Multifactorial Diseases

Non-Mendelian characters are polygenic, meaning that they depend on more than one genetic locus, and they may be multifactorial, with a substantial contribution from environmental as well as genetic factors. Modern medicine recognizes that the diseases that most commonly afflict humans—such as atherosclerosis, hypertension, cancer, diabetes, and arthritis—are multifactorial. The tendency to atherosclerosis, for example, seems to depend on hereditary factors and also on environmental factors such as diet and exercise. There is a great diversity of multifactorial diseases, but a very general explanation schema covers them. Because much research is now taking place into the genetic causes of these diseases, the diseases are increasingly falling into the realm of molecular genetics. In 1996 alone, genetic correlates were identified for such multifactorial diseases as diabetes, pancreatic cancer, and basal cell carcinoma.

Multifactorial Disease Explanation Schema
    Explanation target:
      Why does a **patient** get a **disease** with associated **symptoms**?
    Explanatory pattern:
      The **patient** has inherited various **genes**.

The **patient** is subject to various **environmental factors**.
The **genes** and the **environmental factors** interact to produce the disease.

Although identification of genes relevant to many diseases is proceeding apace, the complex processes by which genes interact with environmental factors are often hard to identify. (The next section on cancer does describe some recent successes, however.) Explanation schemas for particular diseases such as atherosclerosis do not fully describe causal processes but can describe the general causality of disease, as in the following schema:

Atherosclerosis Explanation Schema:

Explanation target:
Why does a **patient** get **atherosclerosis** with associated **symptoms** such as chest pain?

Explanatory pattern:
The **patient** has inherited various **genes** that encourage the development of risk factors such as hyperlipidemia, hypertension, and diabetes.
The **patient** is subject to various **environmental factors**, such as a high-fat diet.
The **genes** and the **environmental factors** interact to produce the disease.

The number and diversity of multifactorial diseases is too great to diagram a hierarchy of multifactorial disease explanation schemas. Medical textbooks usually classify diseases according to the organ system affected, as in diseases of the lungs or of the stomach. Diseases are also classified in terms of type of disease, as in infectious or nutritional diseases. As more is learned about the genetic influences of multifactorial diseases and about the interaction of genetic and environmental factors, new classifications of these diseases should become possible.

Cancer

There are more than one hundred kinds of cancer, and medical professionals including pathologists, epidemiologists, and oncologists have traditionally treated them as diverse diseases. But molecular genetics has made possible a theory of cancer causation that ties these diseases together, as Bishop and Weinberg report (1996, p. 1): "There is now good reason to believe that a unifying explanation for cancer has been found. No matter what form cancer takes, it remains a malady of genes, and most, if not all, causes of cancer act by damaging genes directly or indirectly." Thus, cancer, the second leading cause of death in advanced countries after heart disease, falls under the Molecular Genetics Disease Explanation Schema.

Since the early 1980s, medical research has discovered that cancer is fundamentally a disease of individual cells and that the behavior of cells can be understood in terms of the genes operating within them. Our bodies contain approximately 10^{14} cells, whose frequent divisions offer abundant opportunities for harmful genetic mutations to occur. But it is estimated that six or seven successive mutations are needed to convert a normal cell into an invasive carcinoma (Strachan and Read 1996). The genesis of tumors is a multistep process in which successive damage to various genes leads to different kinds of cancer. Recent research has identified three kinds of genes that are frequently mutated in cancer: oncogenes, tumor suppressor genes, and mutator genes. An oncogene is a gene involved in cell proliferation that can help transform a normal cell into a tumor cell. More than one hundred oncogenes have been identified, such as the E6 and E7 oncogenes found in the human papilloma virus HPV16, which can lead to cervical cancer. Some oncogenes are inserted into cells by viruses, but others are mutated versions of genes that are involved in a variety of normal cellular functions. These normal genes, called *proto-oncogenes*, can be transformed by mutations that produce a gain of function, such as increased production of a protein or production of a modified protein, which leads to the stimulation of cell growth. Causes of such mutations can include environmental factors such as smoking and chemical exposure. But oncogenes alone are not sufficient to produce cancer, because cells contain numerous ways of repairing DNA damage. Tumor suppressor genes produce proteins that constrain cell proliferation and help control the unceasing cell growth that oncogenes can cause. Cancers generally arise when the operation of an oncogene, produced by a virus or a mutation in a proto-oncogene, is followed by mutation in a tumor suppressor gene, which then fails to perform its function of controlling growth. This is called the *two-hit* theory of carcinogenesis. More than a dozen tumor suppressor genes have been discovered, such as BRCA1 and BRCA2 which, when rendered ineffective by mutation, often contribute to breast cancer. Other genes implicated in cancer are mutator genes whose loss of function makes a cell prone to errors in information transfer. The role of various oncogenes and tumor suppressor genes in many human cancers is now well established.

The result of these developments is the following disease schema that provides the unifying explanation advocated by Bishop, Weinberg (1996), and other researchers:

Cancer Explanation Schema

   Explanation target:
      Why does a **patient** get a **cancer?**
   Explanatory pattern:
      The **patient** has **cells** with active **oncogenes** resulting from a viral infection or a mutation of proto-oncogenes.
      These **cells** also contain mutated **tumor suppressor genes.**
      The **tumor suppressor genes** have failed to stop the stimulation of

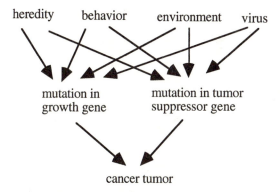

Figure 2.7. Mechanisms of cancer production.
Arrows indicate possible causal relations.

growth in the **cells** produced by the **oncogenes**, generating the **patient's cancer**.

This schema applies to many different cancers, involving different kinds of cells (e.g., those of the lung, breast, or prostate) containing different kinds of oncogenes and tumor suppressor genes. For example, a lung cancer explanation schema would specify the typical process of genetic damage caused by smoking. Cancer is clearly a disease that is both polygenic and multifactorial, involving a number of different genes and various inherited and environmental factors that can contribute to mutations.

Explanation schemas for multifactorial diseases can be vividly depicted using causal network diagrams such as the one in Figure 2.7, which displays how mutations in oncogenes and tumor suppressor genes can arise from various causes and can together produce cancer. Verbal schemas such as the Cancer Explanation Schema and pictorial displays of causal networks such as Figure 2.7 both generate explanations as a matter of fit to a particular situation. To explain why a patient became sick is a matter of finding an explanation schema that fits well with the patient's disease and relevant causal factors such as heredity and environment. To make the fit complete, we need to instantiate the terms in the explanation schema (or, equivalently, the factors in the causal network) to provide an answer to the explanatory target, which concerns why the patient became sick. Instantiation can be based on factors known to apply to a patient, such as smoking, or on factors hypothesized to apply, such as genetic disposition based on the frequent familial occurrence of a particular kind of cancer. See chapter 7 for further discussion of causal explanation.

For example, to explain why Fred, a patient with lung cancer, got his disease, we may be able to construct a causal network like the one in Figure 2.8.

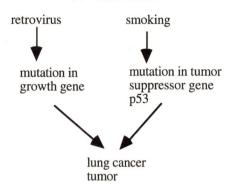

Figure 2.8. Causal explanation of a particular cancer.

This instantiated causal network provides a good fit to Fred's personal situation, although some of the connections in the causal network may be highly conjectural. The explanation of why Fred got cancer does not conform to a deductive or statistical pattern, because there are no universal laws to produce deductions, nor are their sufficient data to provide precise statistical connections between causal factors and carcinogenesis. As with the germ theory, it is difficult to state the new "unifying explanation" extolled by Bishop and Weinberg in terms of universal laws or general models. But the preceding Cancer Explanation Schema captures the kind of causal mechanism that is now believed to be responsible for many different kinds of cancer.

EXPLANATORY AND CONCEPTUAL UNIFICATION

Science is of course much more than a collection of observed facts. In physics, theories such as general relativity and quantum mechanics provide general principles that apply to many phenomena. Evolutionary theory and genetics provide similar unification to biology, as does the theory of plate tectonics to earth science. In medicine, however, unified understanding does not come from the availability of a general overarching theory but from the availability of a system of explanation schemas (these are partly shown in Figure 2.9). Maximum simplicity would result from the applicability of a single explanation schema that accounted for all diseases, as in the eighteenth-century claim by Benjamin Rush that there is only one disease and only one cause: "irregular or convulsive action in the system affected" (quoted in Shryock 1969, p. 3). But as Albert Einstein is reputed to have said, everything should be as simple as possible but not simpler.

My analysis of medical explanation schemas supports the view of Schaffner

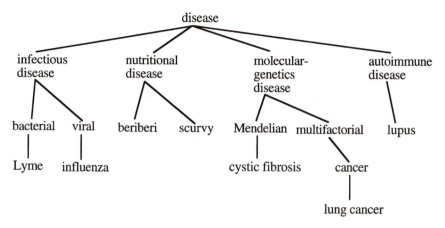

Figure 2.9. Hierarchical organization of disease explanations, with examples of particular diseases. See chapter 10 for further discussion.

(1993) that middle-range biomedical theories are best characterized in terms of hierarchical cognitive structures. These structures provide explanations by fitting particular diseases into general concepts based on common mechanisms. Medical explanation is a matter of fit with causal schemas at different levels of generality, ranging from particular patients to particular diseases to levels of kinds of diseases. Unification in medicine is simultaneously explanatory and conceptual, because what ties explanations together is an organized system of disease concepts.

In recent decades, molecular genetics has made possible new explanation schemas that are having rich applications to Mendelian diseases, cancers, and a wide range of multifactorial diseases that afflict many humans. Chapter 1 argued that the origins of scientific knowledge are also multifactorial and involve a complex of explanation schemas. The next four chapters provide a multifaceted explanation of an important recent development in the theory and treatment of a common disease.

The history of medicine in the nineteenth and twentieth centuries is much richer than my schematic account indicates. Before Pasteur, there were variants of a germ theory of disease as well as a theory that some diseases are caused by miasmas (atmospheric vapors). Much fuller historical treatments include those of Have et al. (1990), Heidel (1941), Hudson (1983), King (1982), Kiple (1993), Magner (1992), Nuland (1988), and Temkin (1973). Philosophical discussions of the nature of disease include the work of Caplan et al. (1981) and Reznek (1987). Also relevant to the germ theory of disease are works on the history of microbiology, such as those by Brock (1961), Collard (1976), Grafe (1991), and Lechevalier and Solotorovsky (1974).

SUMMARY

Disease explanation schemas provide patterns of causal relations responsible for diseases and their symptoms. In the nineteenth century, the humoral theory of disease gave way to the germ theory, which employed different explanation schemas involving infectious agents. Since then, medical research has added explanation schemas for diseases due to nutritional deficiencies, autoimmune reactions, and processes of molecular genetics. Diseases such as cancers can be explained by being fit into a general pattern of genetic and environmental factors. Unified knowledge in medicine comes not from a general set of principles but from the broad applicability of an organized system of explanation schemas.

Part Two

THE BACTERIAL THEORY OF
PEPTIC ULCERS

CHAPTER 3

Ulcers and Bacteria: Discovery

IN 1983, Australian physicians Robin Warren and Barry Marshall reported finding a new kind of bacteria in the stomachs of people with gastritis. Warren and Marshall were soon led to the hypothesis that peptic ulcers are in general caused not by excess acidity or stress but by a bacterial infection. This hypothesis was initially viewed as preposterous, but in 1994 a U.S. National Institutes of Health (NIH) Consensus Development Panel concluded that infection appears to play an important contributory role in the pathogenesis of peptic ulcers and recommended that antibiotics be used in their treatment. Peptic ulcers are common, affecting up to ten percent of the population, and evidence has mounted that many ulcers can be cured by eradicating the bacteria responsible for them.

This chapter is the first of four that discuss the development and reception of the bacterial theory of ulcers from a combination of historical, methodological, psychological, and social perspectives. It examines the nature of the discoveries made by Marshall and Warren, including the new bacteria now known as *Helicobacter pylori*, the hypothesis that peptic ulcers are often the result of bacterial infection, and the hypothesis that peptic ulcers can be cured by treatment with antibiotics. This chapter also describes the kinds of conceptual change that attended the adoption of these hypotheses. The perspective in this chapter is cognitive and considers the mental operations that produced the discovery of the bacterial theory of ulcers. Chapter 4 provides a cognitive account of the acceptance of the new hypotheses.

Chapters 5 and 6 look at the same case from physical and social perspectives. The development of the bacterial theory of ulcers depended on the physical use of instruments such as microscopes and endoscopes and on the devising of experiments to test the association of *H. pylori* and gastric problems. It also had important social dimensions, including the collaborative work of Marshall, Warren, and their associates; the processes of communication by which the new concepts and hypotheses spread; and the processes of negotiation by which consensus began to form (e.g., on the NIH panel). Chapter 6 shows how social explanations of scientific development can complement psychological and methodological explanations. These four chapters together give a broad, integrated, naturalistic explanation of a recent episode in medical science, treating science as a complex system of interacting cognitive, physical, and social processes.

THE DISCOVERIES

Until recently, the stomach was widely believed to be a sterile environment, too acidic for bacteria to survive for long. This acidity is implicated in the common problem of peptic ulcers, sores that can develop in the stomach (gastric ulcers) or below it in the duodenum (duodenal ulcers). Since the 1970s, anti-acid drugs such as cimetidine and ranitidine have been available to provide effective relief from peptic ulcers, although they provide no cure.

During the 1990s, a dramatic shift has occurred in the understanding and treatment of peptic ulcers, leading them to be widely viewed as bacterial in origin and treatable by antibiotics. The shift originated with the work of Warren and Marshall. After sketching the history of the discoveries concerning gastric bacteria and peptic ulcers, I describe four current models of scientific discovery and show how the models contribute to explanation of the three discoveries.

Discovery 1: Helicobacter pylori

In 1979, Robin Warren, a pathologist at Royal Perth Hospital, observed spiral bacteria in a biopsy specimen taken from the stomach of a man with nonulcer dyspepsia (Marshall 1989). Using a microscope, Warren observed severe gastritis as well as microorganisms coating the mucosa (see chapter 5 for details about the use of the microscope). Over the next two years, Warren observed the bacteria in many specimens, which were usually associated with gastritis (Warren and Marshall 1983).

Spiral bacterial had been previously observed in the stomachs of various carnivores, including humans, but they were not viewed as medically significant. In 1981, Barry Marshall began a six-month gastroenterology assignment as part of his training program in internal medicine. The chief of gastroenterology suggested that Marshall help Warren investigate the bacteria he had observed. Warren and Marshall noticed similarities between the gastric spiral bacteria and bacteria of the genus *Campylobacter.* In April 1982, the spiral organism was cultured for the first time. It became apparent that this was a new species of bacteria, which was given the name *Campylobacter pyloridis* in 1983. (The pylorus is the opening from the stomach into the duodenum, which is the first part of the intestine.) In 1987, the name was corrected to *Campylobacter pylori*, but RNA analysis and other studies led to the determination that the bacteria did not belong in the genus *Campylobacter*, and the name was changed again to *Helicobacter pylori* (Goodwin et al. 1989). Several other species of the genus *Helicobacter* are now recognized in ferrets, cats, and dogs. Since 1983, more than three thousand papers have been published on *H. pylori.*

Discovery 2: The Hypothesis that **H. pylori** *Cause Ulcers*

Warren had noticed the association of spiral bacteria with gastritis, but a more controlled study was needed to determine the medical role of *Helicobacter pylori* organisms. Marshall designed a study that measured correlations in one hundred patients between the occurrence of the bacteria and the presence of stomach problems. In his reading on gastritis and bacteria, Marshall found that chronic gastritis was associated with peptic ulcer (Marshall 1989, p. 15). In October 1982, he obtained the statistical results of the study and noticed that only people with gastritis had the gastric spiral bacteria and that all thirteen patients with duodenal ulcer had the organism. In January 1983, Marshall submitted a report for the meeting of the Australian Gastroenterology Society contending that the bacteria may be responsible for ulcers. Although fifty-nine of the sixty-seven submissions for this meeting were accepted, Marshall's was not. Nevertheless, Marshall and Warren published the results of their study in *Lancet*, noting that "the bacteria were present in almost all patients with active chronic gastritis, duodenal ulcer, or gastric ulcer and thus may be an important factor in the aetiology of these diseases" (Marshall and Warren 1984, p. 1311).

Although many gastroenterologists initially viewed the hypothesis that peptic ulcers are caused by bacteria as preposterous, subsequent studies have strongly supported the claim of Marshall and Warren, and the hypothesis is now largely accepted by gastroenterologists. Chapter 4 reviews the considerations that affected the initial rejection of the hypothesis that *H. pylori* causes ulcers and its subsequent widespread acceptance.

Discovery 3: Peptic Ulcers Can Be Treated with Antibiotics

In medical research, discoveries often have practical as well as theoretical importance. In 1981, before their systematic study had even begun, Marshall and Warren prescribed tetracycline treatment for a man with severe gastric discomfort caused by gastritis. After fourteen days of antibiotics, the gastritis and the discomfort were gone. Marshall had read that recurrence rates for ulcers were reduced by treatment with bismuth citrate (e.g., the over-the-counter drug Pepto-Bismol) and found that the bismuth preparation De-Nol had an inhibitory affect on *H. pylori* in vitro. Subsequent clinical trials determined that a combination of metronidazole and bismuth eradicated *H. pylori* infection in eighty precent of patients, and various similar therapies have also been found to be effective (D. Y. Graham 1995, 1996; Marshall 1994). Eradication produces duodenal ulcer cure rates of ninety percent; cure rates are lower for gastric ulcers, thirty-five percent of which are caused not by bacteria but by nonsteroidal anti-inflammatory drugs such as aspirin.

MODELS OF DISCOVERY

To understand cognitive aspects of these three discoveries, we can look to four models of discovery that have been influential in philosophical, psychological, and computational research on scientific thinking. What were the cognitive processes that produced Marshall and Warren's discoveries? I consider four models of discovery processes: search, questioning, blind variation, and serendipity.

Discovery as Search

In computational and psychological work on scientific discovery, the most prevalent model uses the notion of search in a space of possibilities. This model originated in Newell and Simon's (1972) theory of problem solving as involving a set of states and a set of operators for moving from state to state. Search is the process of finding a sequence of operators that leads from the initial state of knowledge to the goal state in which the problem is solved. Heuristics are rules of thumb that make the search intelligently selective rather than random. Search through a problem space is an excellent way to characterize well-defined problems such as playing chess, and it also applies to discovery problems such as finding mathematical laws that describe given data (Langley et al. 1987).

Schunn and Klahr (1995) have proposed a model of discovery that involves search in four spaces. They write (p. 106):

> One fruitful characterization of scientific discovery is to view it in terms of search in two problem spaces: a space of hypotheses and a space of experiments (Klahr & Dunbar 1988; Simon & Lea 1974). . . . In [Schunn and Klahr's] new framework, what has been previously conceived as the *hypothesis space* has now been divided into a *data representation space* and a *hypothesis space*. In the hypothesis space, hypotheses about causal relations in the data are drawn using the set of features in the current representation. Similarly, the old *experiment space* is now divided into an *experimental paradigm space* and an *experiment space*. In the experimental paradigm space, a class of experiments (i.e., a paradigm) is chosen which identifies the factors to vary, and the components which are held constant. In the experiment space, the parameter settings within the selected paradigm are chosen.

New data representations can be produced by learning mechanisms such as concept formation and analogy (Holland et al. 1986). The search model of hypothesis discovery is summarized in the following explanation schema, which is similar to the Cognitive Explanation Schema for belief acquisition (chapter 1):

Search Explanation Schema

Explanation target:

Why did a **scientist** discover a **hypothesis**?

Explanatory pattern:

The **scientist** had **mental representations** that established a **search space** of possible hypotheses.

The **scientist** had **mental procedures** for using the **search space** to generate new hypotheses.

The **scientist's** search generated the **hypothesis**.

Discovery as Questioning

But search may not be the best way to describe discoveries by scientists who do not have well-defined problems, goals, or operators. Kleiner (1993) describes how Charles Darwin's discovery of evolution by natural selection was guided by a series of questions, such as the following:

Q1. Do species transmute?

Q2. Are Galapagos specimens distinct species or distinct varieties?

Q3. Do the variations observable among the mockingbird specimens correspond to variations among acknowledged species?

Questions Q3 and Q2 are relevant to Q1, which also gave rise to the question of *how* species transmute, a question that was eventually answered by the theory of natural selection. Darwin's intellectual problem, however, was much too complex and ill-defined for us to specify a problem space in terms of states and operators, but we can nevertheless understand the development of his views in terms of a series of questions that he posed to himself. Various writers in philosophy, psychology, and artificial intelligence have emphasized the importance of question generation and answering to the process of inquiry (Bromberger 1992; Hintikka and Vandamme 1985; Lauer, et al. 1992; Ram 1991).

Where do new scientific questions come from? Some are generated as subordinate questions designed to answer questions already posed. Truly original questions seem to arise from three major sources: surprise, practical need, and curiosity. Surprise occurs when something is found that is not coherent with previous expectations and beliefs, for example, when Darwin found an unusual distribution of species in the Galapagos. Practical need generates scientific questions when the accomplishment of some technological task is seen to require additional knowledge about how the world works, as when the Manhattan project gave rise to questions in atomic physics crucial to building an atomic bomb. Curiosity generates questions when there is something that a scientist wants to know out of general interest, not because of previous surprise or practical need. Here are patterns for four kinds of scientific question generation:

A. *Surprise*
  1. A scientist is surprised to learn information that does not cohere with existing knowledge.
  2. The scientist therefore asks for an explanation of the information.

B. *Need*
  1. A scientist has practical goals (e.g., medical or technological goals).
  2. The scientist is not aware of any means to accomplish these goals.
  3. The scientist therefore asks how to accomplish the goals.

C. *Curiosity*
  1. A scientist has considerable knowledge about a phenomenon, P1.
  2. There is a phenomenon, P2, which is similar to P1, but many kinds of information available about P1 are not available about P2.
  3. The scientist therefore asks questions about P2 with potential answers similar to what is known about P1.

D. *Subordinate questions*
  1. A scientist wants to answer a question Q1.
  2. Answering question Q2 is relevant to answering Q1, because one of the following holds time:
      (a) The answer to Q2 entails the answer to Q1.
      (b) The answer to Q2 might provide evidence relevant to an answer to Q1;
      (c) The answer to Q2 is analogically relevant to an answer to Q1, because Q2 and Q1 are similar questions.

Undoubtedly, this is not an exhaustive set of ways of generating scientific questions, but it will be useful for discussing discoveries about ulcers and bacteria. Discovery as questioning yields the following cognitive explanation schema:

Questioning Explanation Schema
  Explanation target:
    Why did a **scientist** discover a **hypothesis**?
  Explanatory pattern:
    The **scientist** had **mental representations** of **questions** arising from surprise, need, or curiosity.
    The **scientist** had **mental procedures** for generating answers to **questions**, including the generation of subordinate questions.
    The **scientist's** attempt to answer questions generated the **hypothesis**.

Discovery as Blind Variation

Search and questioning are both heuristic methods in which considerable knowledge is used to guide discovery. Campbell (1988) and others have argued, in contrast, that discoveries arise because of a process of blind variation akin to what occurs in genetic mutation. These proponents of evolutionary epistemology have defended a biological model of discovery in which hypotheses are formed by blind variation or recombination, just as biological organisms achieve genetic diversity through mutation and chromosomal crossover. Computer scientists have devised powerful genetic algorithms modeled on mutation and recombination (Holland 1975; Koza 1992). There is, however, no psychological or neurological evidence that such algorithms are part of human cognition. For a more favorable view of evolutionary epistemology, see Cziko (1996); for critiques, see Thagard (1988 [chapter 8] and 1992b [chapter 6]).

Discovery as Serendipity

Many discoveries in science are accidental, in that they come about in ways that were not planned by the scientists who made them. Roberts (1989) distinguishes between *serendipity*, which describes accidental discoveries of things not sought for, and *pseudoserendipity*, which describes accidental discoveries of ways to achieve an end sought for. Charles Goodyear's discovery of the vulcanization of rubber, which occurred when he accidentally dropped a piece of rubber mixed with sulfur onto a hot stove, was pseudoserendipity, since he had been searching for a way to make rubber useful for years. Similarly, Alexander Fleming's discovery of penicillin came after years of investigations into antibacterial compounds, but his discovery that *Penicillium* mold can kill bacteria was accidental. In contrast, when George deMestral invented Velcro after noticing how burrs stuck to his dog, it was serendipity, since he was not looking for a new fastener. Wilhelm Röntgen's discovery of x-rays was similarly serendipitous, as he was not looking for new kinds of radiation. Antony van Leeuwenhoek was merely trying to soften pepper when he accidentally discovered bacteria (see chapter 10). Serendipity in this sense is not well characterized as *search*, since there is no problem to be solved. Pseudoserendipity is also not well characterized as search, since the solution comes about by accidental introduction of an operator (e.g., dropping the rubber on the stove) that was not part of the initial problem space. Comroe (1977) provides numerous examples of serendipity in medical discovery, including cases in which chance helped scientists reach their committed goals, and ones in which chance changed their goals and set them in new directions.

Integrating the Four Models

These four models of discovery are not competing theories, for they highlight potentially complementary aspects of the process of scientific discovery. Discovery as blind variation can be included within the model of discovery as search, if blind variation is seen as a nonheuristic search strategy. From a computational perspective, blind variation seems likely to be slow and ineffective: Cognition operates much more efficiently than biological evolution, which has myriad organisms and vast stretches of time. In current computational work on genetic algorithms, the most powerful operation is not mutation but crossover, in which two strong representations are combined.

Advocates of the search model of discovery will likely argue that questioning can also be assimilated to search. Perhaps one could posit a "question space" to expand further Schunn and Klahr's (1995) four-space model, arguing that researchers first search the question space and then move on to explore the other four spaces. But the putative question space, like their data representation and experimental paradigm spaces, is so vast and ill defined that I see little explanatory gain in describing it as being searched. The metaphor of discovery as search applies well to a hypothesis space in which the representations are given and to an experimental space in which the paradigms are given, but the metaphor becomes unacceptably vague when stretched to cover uncharted territory.

Schunn and Klahr's expanded model also assumes, like the standard search model, that discoverers are working with a problem that was presented to them. It does not address the issue of problem generation, which is the same as the issue of how potentially fertile questions arise. So the formation of interesting questions should not be assimilated to the search model. But questioning and search *are* related, in that the formulation of even vague questions can lead toward defining problems that can be solved by search. Once a question is formulated, subordinate questions relevant to answering can be suggested, and it may be possible to answer some of these by solving well-defined problems in a fashion appropriately characterized as search. Hence the Search Explanation Schema and the Questioning Explanation Schema can be complementary.

Similarly, serendipity may contribute to both questioning and search. Serendipity may provide a surprising or curiosity-inducing event that inspires questioning, as when Newton's perception of the fall of an apple moved him to wonder why objects fall toward the earth's center. Moreover, when a search is underway, serendipity may provide a representation or operator that was not part of the original problem space, as when Goodyear discovered vulcanization. Kantorovich (1993) views serendipity as a kind of blind variation but is vague about what is varied. Ignoring blind variation, Figure 3.1 shows the influence relations of serendipity, questioning, and search. Questioning arises

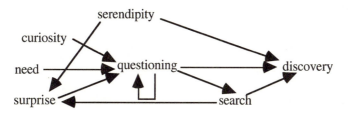

Figure 3.1. Interrelations of models of discovery

from curiosity, need, surprise, or a combination of these and can lead to discovery, search, or more questioning. Surprise can arise from serendipity or from the results of search. Discovery can be the result of various combinations of serendipity, questioning, and search. Let us now see how these models help explain the three discoveries concerning bacteria and ulcers.

MODELING THE DISCOVERIES

Discovery 1: **Helicobacter pylori**

The discovery of *H. pylori* and the formation of the hypothesis that these bacteria routinely colonize human stomachs were the result of a combination of serendipity, questioning, and search. Warren's initial noticing of the spiral gastric bacteria can best be described as serendipitous. He was not seeking an explanation of gastritis or ulcers, and he just happened to examine gastric specimens with sufficient magnification to make bacteria visible. Warren was not consciously following up on the research of others who had observed similar bacteria (e.g., Fung et al. 1979; Steer and Colin-Jones 1975). Steer and Colin-Jones (1975) had reported finding bacteria in gastric epithelium and observed the correlation of these bacteria with gastric ulceration, but they misidentified them as *Pseudomonas aeruginosa.* Warren independently and accidentally discovered the bacteria in the course of his everyday work. Persistent in the face of colleagues who were skeptical about the bacteria, he pursued a more systematic observation of the bacteria.

Serendipity also played a role in efforts to culture the bacteria. During the 1970s, techniques for culturing *Campylobacter* had been developed, but thirty attempts in late 1981 to use these techniques to culture the gastric bacteria failed in part, it was later discovered, because of faulty incubators. Agar plates on which the bacteria were supposed to grow had been discarded after forty-eight hours with no visible growth. Then in April 1982, because of a four-day Easter weekend and other demands on the microbiology laboratory, the culture was left in the incubator for five days, long enough for bacterial colonies to become visible (Marshall 1989, p. 14). This event is an example of pseudoserendipity, since the investigators certainly had the goal of culturing the bacteria, but incubating for five days was not a method they had been considering.

Surprise and curiosity led Warren to ask questions about the nature of these bacteria, and he requested a silver stain that made the number and shape of the microorganisms much more evident. Surprise was certainly a factor, since it was generally believed that the stomach is sterile. Curiosity was piqued by the fact that little was known about the stomach bacteria, in contrast to the vast amount of information available concerning other bacteria. Marshall joined in the questioning about the nature of the bacteria, stating in his part of the letter to *Lancet:* "The above description of S-shaped spiral bacteria in the gastric antrum, by my colleague Dr. J. R. Warren, raises the following questions: why have they not been seen before; are they pathogens or merely commensals in a damaged mucosa; and are they campylobacters?" (Warren and Marshall 1983, p. 1273). Marshall engaged in a systematic literature search to try to find out whether they were members of an already known species. Thus, the question, "What are these bacteria?" gave rise to a fairly well-defined search to answer the question, "Are these bacteria of any known species?" The answer to that question turned out to be negative, so initially a new species and eventually a new genus, *Helicobacter*, were generated. In the terms of Schunn and Klahr, this discovery would be described as the result of a search through a space of representations, but that space is so ill-defined that the relevance of the search metaphor is dubious. Marshall (1989, p. 16), reported the following:

> For me, identification of the bacterium posed a problem. None of the textbooks gave details concerning where to start when totally new bacteria are discovered. Most books merely told how to test if a bacterium was the same as, or different from, the known species. In a clinical laboratory this meant checking a new isolate against a panel of known pathogens and then discarding it if no match was made.

The question of the nature of bacteria inspired a search for identification with known bacteria, but the failure of this search required the postulation of a new species.

In sum, the discovery of *H. pylori* is best described as the result of serendipity and surprise. These elements produced questioning that led to a search, and the search produced more questioning that generated the recognition of a new species of bacteria.

Discovery 2: The Hypothesis that Helicobacter pylori *Bacteria Cause Ulcers*

Although the existence of *H. pylori* in the human stomach was quickly accepted by gastroenterologists and microbiologists, the etiological role of these bacteria remained contentious into the 1990s (see chapter 4). A skeptic would write of the discovery of the *hypothesis* that bacteria cause ulcers rather than of the discovery *that* bacteria cause ulcers. Marshall concluded his 1983 letter: "If these bacteria are truly associated with antral gastritis, as described by Warren, they may have a part to play in other poorly understood, gastritis associated diseases (i.e., peptic ulcer and gastric cancer)" (Warren and Marshall 1983, p. 1274). How did the conjecture that the bacteria may cause ulcers arise?

The first step in the generation of this hypothesis was Warren's observation of an association between the gastric spiral bacteria and gastritis. This association was obvious to him from his first observations of the bacteria: In the biopsies he was examining, it was clear that stomach cells close to the bacteria were damaged, whereas cells remote from the bacteria were not. From Warren's perspective, observation immediately suggested a causal connection between the bacteria and stomach inflammation. But his attempts to interest gastroenterologists in the bacteria were unsuccessful until Marshall was assigned to do a research project with him.

As a practicing physician, Marshall naturally raised the question of whether the newly discovered bacteria were pathogens. This question is inspired not merely by curiosity but also by the professional need to treat illnesses. Marshall was aware that many stomach problems such as gastritis and ulcers could be reduced but not generally cured by antacids. The question, "Are the bacteria pathogenic?" could be made more specific: "What gastric diseases might the bacteria produce?" Because there are only a relatively small number of such diseases, it was possible to search for disease correlates of the bacteria. The search took two forms, literary and experimental. During his extensive reading in the summer of 1982, Marshall encountered the repeated observation that chronic gastritis was associated with peptic ulcer (Marshall 1989, p. 15). He already knew from Warren's work that gastritis and bacteria were associated. So it was natural to consider that the bacteria might be associated with peptic ulcer. Marshall designed a study aiming to "(1) decide if the bacteria were associated with gastritis, (2) find the source of infection, (3) culture the bacteria, and (4) determine which diseases, if any, were associated with infection" (Marshall 1989, p. 13). The study conducted in 1982 looked for associations between stomach appearance as judged by endoscopy and the occurrence of bacteria as indicated by biopsy. Bacteria were found in 77% of patients with gastric ulcers and in 100% of patients with duodenal ulcer, in contrast to 50% of patients with normal stomachs (Marshall and Warren 1984, p. 1312).

Marshall's formation of the hypothesis that spiral bacteria cause ulcers thus depended on the following chain of associations:

1. Bacteria are associated with gastritis (Warren).
2. Gastritis is associated with ulcers (reading).
3. Bacteria may therefore be associated with ulcers.

4. Bacteria are associated with ulcers (experimental study).
5. Bacteria may therefore cause ulcers.

Marshall and Warren (1984, p. 1314) concluded their paper by saying: "Although cause-and-effect cannot be proved in a study of this kind, we believe that pyloric campylobacter is aetiologically related to chronic gastritis, and, probably, to peptic ulceration also." The inference from step 4 to step 5 seems to derive from a simple heuristic: *If A and B are associated with each other, then they may be causally related.* Once the search for associates of the bacteria turned up ulcers, the leap to considering a possible causal relation was automatic. Could it be, on the other hand, that ulcers cause bacteria by virtue of a stomach ulcer providing a fertile environment for bacteria to grow? Given the occurrence of bacteria in patients without ulcers and the fact that the bacteria were not found to be prominent on gastric ulcer borders, it was more plausible that bacteria cause ulcers than vice versa.

Thus, the process of discovering the hypothesis that ulcers are caused by bacteria included questioning leading to search and application of a heuristic to infer causality from association. Since the pioneering work of Marshall and Warren, *H. pylori* has also been implicated as a possible cause of stomach cancer, dyspepsia, and heart disease. Establishing that a correlated factor is indeed a cause is an extremely complex process that is discussed in chapters 4 and 7.

Discovery 3: Peptic Ulcers Can Be Treated with Antibiotics

Although bacteria were observed by Leeuwenhoek as early as 1676, their role in disease was not appreciated until after 1860, when Pasteur, Lister, Koch, and others showed that such diseases as tuberculosis have bacterial causes (see chapter 2). Antibiotic treatments that cure disease by eliminating the responsible bacteria became available only in the 1940s. For Warren and Marshall, however, the germ theory of disease and antibiotic treatments were utterly familiar, so it is not surprising that as early as 1981 they treated a gastritis patient with tetracycline. The question of whether ulcers could be cured with antibiotics may have arisen analogically:

1. Ulcers are associated with and may be caused by bacteria.
2. Similarly infectious diseases (e.g., tuberculosis) caused by bacteria can be cured by antibiotics.
3. Therefore, perhaps ulcers can also be cured by antibiotics.

The question of whether ulcers can be cured by antibiotics converted immediately into a search for what antibiotics are most effective. Given the extensive knowledge about treatment of bacterial infections available by the 1980s, this problem was relatively well defined and the search quite manageable. Marshall

(1994) describes various regimens that are effective for eradicating *H. pylori* and curing many cases of peptic ulcers.

The three discoveries about ulcers and bacteria therefore varied in the extent of the roles played by serendipity, questioning, and search. Serendipity played a large role in the discovery of the spiral bacteria, whereas questioning seems to have been most important to the formation of the hypothesis that bacteria cause ulcers, and search sufficed to find successful antibiotic treatments for ulcers.

CONCEPTUAL CHANGE

The three discoveries so far discussed can all be framed as propositions: the discovery that stomachs contain spiral bacteria, that ulcers are caused by bacteria, and that ulcers can be treated with antibiotics. But the growth of scientific knowledge is not simply a matter of generating new hypotheses. It also involves the introduction of new concepts and the alteration of existing ones. Medical researchers and other scientists sometimes use *concept* to mean *hypothesis*; but by concepts I mean mental representations correlative to words such as *ulcer* and *bacteria*, in contrast to propositions correlative to whole sentences such as "Bacteria cause ulcers." Thagard (1992b) showed that seven major scientific revolutions—those of Copernicus, Newton, Einstein, Lavoisier, and Darwin, and development of the quantum theory and the theory of plate tectonics—all involved substantial conceptual change.

The two kinds of conceptual change most relevant to the ulcer/bacteria case are concept formation and reclassification. *Concept formation* involves the generation of new concepts such as the mental representation of a new species of bacteria, whereas *reclassification* involves revision in the kind relations that organize concepts in mental systems. In cognitive psychology, psycholinguistics, and artificial intelligence, it is widely agreed that conceptual systems are structured in large part by kind relations: A robin is a kind of bird which is a kind of animal which is a kind of thing. Reclassification involves moving a concept from one branch in the tree of concepts to another branch.

Undoubtedly, the most important concept formed during the development of knowledge about ulcers and bacteria was the concept of *H. pylori*, and we have already seen that the formation of this concept was historically complex. Warren and Marshall did not simply observe a host of bacteria and dub them with the name *Helicobacter pylori*. They initially used the informal term "gastric spiral bacteria," thus forming a concept by combining existing well-established concepts. The process of conceptual combination is sometimes intersective, producing a new concept that involves the intersection of existing concepts: Spiral bacteria are just bacteria that are spiral (see Thagard 1988 for a discussion of this kind of conceptual combination as a mechanism of discovery). But other conceptual combinations produce puzzlement that leads to emergent properties. Kunda et al. (1990) presented subjects with surprising examples such as "blind lawyer" and found that combination often involved generation of aspects not part of the original concepts; for example, a blind lawyer may be hypothesized to be courageous to explain how someone who is blind could become a lawyer. The conceptual combination "gastric bacteria" is of just this sort, since before Warren's work it was widely believed that the stomach was too acidic for bacterial colonization. Hence the new combination provoked the question: "How can bacteria live in the stomach?" The interesting answer is that members of *H. pylori* bury themselves beneath the mucosal layer and produce ammonia, which neutralizes the gastric acid. The anomalous combination "gastric bacteria" therefore led to an emergent property; that of producing ammonia.

Initially, Warren and Marshall thought that the gastric spiral bacteria might be members of a known species of the genus *Campylobacter*. Had this been so, no concept formation would have been necessary, since the newly discovered objects would have been assimilated to an existing concept. Concept formation often involves differentiation, in which an object or substance is distinguished from ones already conceptualized. Once it became clear that the gastric bacteria did not fall under any known species, it was appropriate to differentiate them under the heading of *Campylobacter pylori*.

From the start, however, it was clear that the flagellar morphology of the gastric bacteria—several sheathed flagella at one end—differed from that of members of the genus *Campylobacter*, which have a single unsheathed flagellum at one or both ends (Marshall and Warren 1984). RNA analysis and other studies eventually showed that the new bacteria are sufficiently distinct from campylobacters to warrant assignation to a new genus, *Helicobacter*. Conceptual change thus involved the formation of new concepts for the genus *Helicobacter* and the species *Helicobacter pylori* as well as reclassification of the new species as *Helicobacter* rather than as *Campylobacter*.

Reclassification of diseases is required for acceptance of the hypothesis that ulcers are caused by bacteria. Marshall remarked that "the *C. pylori* story will mature, in my opinion, when medical texts have a chapter on peptic ulcer disease within the infectious disease section" (Marshall 1989, pp. 20–21). Current medical textbooks organize their discussions of diseases in two parallel ways: in terms of the organ system affected (e.g., cardiovascular diseases, respiratory diseases) and in terms of pathogenesis (e.g., infectious diseases, oncology). The hypothesis that ulcers are caused by bacteria requires reclassification of the disease as an infectious disease, whereas previously it was viewed as caused by acid imbalance or even classified as psychosomatic. Reclassification of ulcers as an infectious disease goes hand in hand with the decision to treat ulcers with antibiotics. Because of the link with *H. pylori*, peptic ulcers now fit the Germ Theory Explanation Schema presented in chapter 2.

Ulcers can be further classified in terms of how various types are caused: "We now recognize at least three types of duodenal ulcer disease: *H. pylori*–related, NSAID [nonsteroidal anti-inflammatory drug-associated, and hypersecretory" (D. Y. Graham 1991a, p. 108). Thus, ulcers can now be viewed as consisting of several kinds, including the kind associated with bacterial infection. Accepting a bacterial cause for most ulcers enabled the reclassification of ulcers as an infectious disease but also required the subdividing of ulcers into infectious and noninfectious types. The concept of *Helicobacter pylori* has also been subject to subcategorization, since two different strains have been suggested, one of them more likely to produce a peptic ulcer than the other (Monmaney 1993).

The discovery of *H. pylori* also led to a change in the concept of gastritis. Marshall (1989, p. 16) said of the 1982 study: "It then became clear that only people with gastritis had the gastric spiral bacteria. We therefore had an association between the bacterium and a condition that was at the time not even recognized as a disease." Previously, gastritis was considered to be so common and to have so many possible causes that it was not considered to be a disease. Once a specific bacterial cause was identified, however, it became possible to reclassify histological gastritis as a bacterial disease. Warren and Marshall's advocacy of such a reclassification still encounters resistance from some gastroenterologists. Chapter 12 provides an account of current controversies concerning the role of *H. pylori* in dyspepsia.

Although appreciation of the bacterial theory of ulcers requires the construction and reorganization of concepts, it would be a gross exaggeration to suggest that the new theory of ulcers was so radically different from the old one that their rational comparison was impossible. According to Kuhn (1970), competing paradigms may be "incommensurable" with each other and their proponents may "live in different worlds." But critics of Warren and Marshall did not have trouble understanding the claim about ulcer causation; the critics just considered the claim to be wrong, or at least undemonstrated. Once evidence accumulated in support of the claim, its acceptance became widespread (see chapter 4). Chapter 10 provides a more general account of conceptual change in medicine.

THE PROCESS OF DISCOVERY

Some philosophical and computational discussions operate with a simplistic model of discovery as the generation of hypotheses from data, as shown in Figure 3.2. Figure 3.1 provided a more realistic model that displayed the roles of serendipity and questioning in scientific discovery in addition to the role of discovery algorithms that govern search. The patterns through which questions are generated by surprise, need, curiosity, and subordinate questions (see

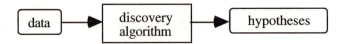

Figure 3.2. Discovery as the generation of hypotheses from data.

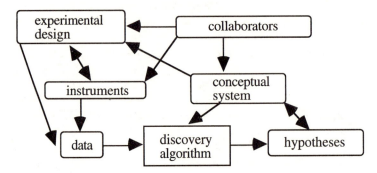

Figure 3.3. Discovery as a complex cognitive, physical, and social process.

earlier in this chapter) are only the beginning of a theory of scientific question generation. Ideally, these patterns should be translated into algorithms that provide a computational model of how scientists generate questions. The ambition of this chapter, however, is more modest: to show how questioning, search, and serendipity all contributed to discoveries about stomach bacteria and ulcers.

Of course, the process of discovery is much more complex than either Figure 3.1 or Figure 3.2 presents. The growth of knowledge about ulcers and bacteria was not just a matter of generation of hypotheses, but it also required considerable conceptual change, including both the formation of new concepts and the reclassification of existing ones. Conceptual systems interact with discovery algorithms in ways suggested by Figure 3.3, which also points to the physical role of instruments and experiments (see chapter 5) and to the social role of collaboration (see chapters 6 and 11). Moreover, the generation of hypotheses is not equivalent to their acceptance, since alternative explanations must be considered (see chapter 4).

SUMMARY

Development of the bacterial theory of ulcers involved three major discoveries: the existence of *H. pylori*, the hypothesis that these bacteria cause peptic ulcers, and the treatment of ulcers with antibiotics. These discoveries involved cognitive processes of questioning and search as well as serendipity. This case also involved substantial conceptual change, including the formation of new concepts such as the mental representation of *H. pylori* and the reclassification of bacteria and diseases. The process of discovery, however, is physical and social as well as cognitive.

CHAPTER 4

Ulcers and Bacteria: Acceptance

WHAT CAUSES peptic ulcers? Medical researchers rarely put the question so starkly, discussing instead various factors in the etiology or pathogenesis of gastric and duodenal ulcers. Between 1983 and 1995, there occurred a dramatic shift in medical beliefs about the causes of ulcers: Most researchers and practicing gastroenterologists concluded that the major factor in peptic ulcers is infection by bacteria of the newly discovered species *Helicobacter pylori*. Chapter 3 identified three hypotheses that have been central to the development of the bacterial theory of ulcers and discussed the cognitive mechanisms responsible for their discovery:

> Hypothesis 1: Gastric spiral bacteria (*H. pylori*) inhabit the human stomach.
> Hypothesis 2: These bacteria can cause peptic ulcers.
> Hypothesis 3: Peptic ulcers can be cured with antibiotics.

I now discuss how these hypotheses have been evaluated by medical researchers and why they have become increasingly accepted.

The two central questions are (1) how the cause of a disease can be ascertained by medical research and (2) how researchers can change their minds about what causes a disease. Barry Marshall and Robin Warren's (1984) suggestion that ulcers may be caused by bacteria was initially viewed by some researchers as absurd and outrageous. Martin Blaser of the Division of Infectious Diseases at the Vanderbilt University School of Medicine thought a 1983 talk by Marshall was "the most preposterous thing I'd ever heard; I thought, This guy is a madman" (Monmaney 1993, p. 65). Blaser (1989; see also Cover and Blaser 1992) has since become one of the leading researchers on *H. pylori*. David Forman of the Imperial Cancer Research Fund thought that Marshall's claim that bacteria are responsible for various stomach diseases, including cancer, was a "totally crazy hypothesis" (Suzuki 1995, p. 9). But he thought it worth demolishing and has since concluded that *H. pylori* infection is a major factor in gastric cancer and in ulcers (Forman et al. 1991; EUROGAST Study Group 1993). Other gastroenterologists were skeptical of Marshall and Warren's claims but were sufficiently intrigued to launch their own research programs.

I will try to explain why the hypotheses about ulcers and bacteria seemed crazy to many in 1983 but why Marshall and Warren nevertheless accepted them. I first describe Marshall's early attempts to convince others of the causal role of *H. pylori* using Koch's postulates, a time-honored method of establishing particular bacteria as causes of a particular disease. Koch's postulates require that the bacteria be transmitted to an uninfected animal and produce disease in it; the postulates have been fulfilled for gastritis but not for ulcers. I identify the causal reasoning that underlies application of Koch's postulates and argue that the postulates are a sufficient but far from necessary means of establishing causality. In addition to a large amount of correlational evidence linking the ulcers and bacteria, numerous experiments have shown that peptic ulcers can be cured by antibiotics. Acceptance of hypothesis 3, that antibiotics cure peptic ulcers, provides major support for hypothesis 2, that ulcers are caused by bacteria. Accepting that bacteria cause ulcers is a major part of the belief change experienced by many medical researchers in the decade between 1985 and 1995, but other interconnected beliefs are also involved. The shift to the bacterial theory of ulcers can be understood in terms of an account of explanatory coherence that has been widely applied to conceptual revolutions in the natural sciences.

EARLY RECEPTION OF THE BACTERIAL THEORY
OF ULCERS

By 1983, after an experiment involving one hundred patients tested for presence of the bacterium and presence of stomach disease; Marshall (1989, p. 19) was convinced that the new bacterium was the primary cause of peptic ulcer disease. All thirteen patients with duodenal ulcer had the bacterium, and the association between gastric ulcers and the bacterium was statistically significant (Marshall and Warren 1984). Marshall was relatively new to gastroenterology, having only begun specialized training in the field in 1981. At the time, his primary interest was in internal medicine, and he had much more experience with infectious diseases than with ulcers. Accordingly, his adoption of the new hypotheses did not require abandonment of a set of well-entrenched beliefs that conflicted with the new ideas. In contrast, other more established medical researchers and practitioners had beliefs about the nature and treatment of ulcers that clashed with the new hypotheses and led them to reject the hypotheses summarily.

Hypothesis 1, that members of a previously unidentified species of bacteria inhabit the human stomach, was initially greeted with incredulity because of prevailing beliefs about the stomach. According to Blaser (1989, pp. 1–2), "most physicians believed that the normal human stomach, because of its high acid concentration, was sterile except for transient bacterial flora." Hypothesis

1, however, was quickly established as numerous researchers who had specialized in research on *Campylobacter* infections in humans turned their attention to what was taken to be a new species of that genus. The new bacteria could be microscopically observed using the staining techniques introduced by Warren, and they could be grown in the laboratory using the culturing techniques developed by Marshall. The apparent conflict between the acidic nature of the stomach and the existence there of bacteria has been resolved by discoveries about the nature of *H. pylori.* These bacteria are able to burrow beneath the mucous layer in the stomach, and they produce an enzyme, urease, that uses urea present in the gastric juice to generate ammonia, an alkaline substance that neutralizes acid (Marshall et al. 1990). Bacteriologists were therefore quick to accept the hypothesis that a newly recognized kind of bacteria inhabit the human stomach.

Many gastroenterologists, however, found it much more difficult to consider a challenge to accepted views about the causes of peptic ulcers. By the early 1980s, it was widely believed that excess stomach acid was the main cause of peptic ulcers. People with increased amounts of acid were found to be more likely to get the disease, and cimetidine (Tagamet) and ranitidine (Zantac) were found to be effective antacid means of healing ulcers. Physicians thus had an explanation in terms of excess acidity of why some people get ulcers as well as an effective means of treating those people (i.e., with cimetidine and ranitidine, which remain among the most widely prescribed drugs). Hence, hypothesis 2—that ulcers are caused by bacteria—clashed with the hypothesis that acidity is the main culprit in peptic ulceration, and hypothesis 3 clashed with the effective standard treatment. It is not surprising, then, that many gastroenterologists rejected the new hypotheses as incoherent with what was already known (see later). As a result, Marshall, a young, unknown Australian who put forward his new hypotheses with confidence amounting to brashness, was viewed as crazy.

In retrospect, there were problems with the accepted view of ulcers. It was not known *why* some people have excess acidity, although conjectures were made about genetic factors and psychological factors such as stress. The popular view of ulcers as a psychosomatic, stress-induced disease had given way to the emphasis on excess acidity, but stress remained one possible indirect explanation of ulcers, since it was known that stomach acid secretion increases in animals under stress. Even more important, although antacid drugs were usually effective in controlling the symptoms of ulcers, it was well known that the recurrence of ulcers was common: The drugs clearly did not produce a cure. Hence, when Marshall began to develop alternative hypotheses about the causes and treatment of ulcers, some researchers took them seriously enough to test them. Marshall, Warren, and their collaborators undertook the task of accumulating evidence concerning the cause and treatment of ulcers.

CAUSATION AND KOCH'S POSTULATES

In 1882, Robert Koch published his discovery of the bacteria that cause tuberculosis, describing his findings that the presence of the tubercle bacillus is strongly correlated with the occurrence and development of the disease. He added that to prove tuberculosis is brought about by the bacilli, the bacilli must be isolated from the body, cultured, and used to transfer the disease to other animals (Brock 1961, p. 111). Koch's requirements for tuberculosis were codified by his colleague Loeffler, who produced the following conditions for demonstrating the parasitic nature of a disease (Brock 1988, p. 180):

1. The parasitic organism must be shown to be constantly present in characteristic form and arrangement in the diseased tissue.

2. The organism, which from its behavior appears to be responsible for the disease, must be isolated and grown in pure culture.

3. The pure culture must be shown to induce the disease experimentally.

Variants of these postulates have been used by generations of microbiologists as a description of what is required to demonstrate that a microorganism is the cause of a disease.

By 1984, Marshall and Warren had satisfied postulates 1 and 2, having shown a strong correlation between *H. pylori* infection and both gastritis and peptic ulcer. But initial attempts to satisfy postulate 3 using pigs were unsuccessful, so Marshall decided to experiment on himself. After undergoing endoscopy to show that he was free of gastric disease, he swallowed a flourishing three-day culture of the bacteria. After a week, he vomited and developed putrid breath, and biopsy showed that he had gastritis and his stomach contained the spiral bacteria (Marshall et al. 1985). Hence Koch's postulates had been fulfilled to establish that *H. pylori* infection causes gastritis. Since then, Koch's third postulate has also been satisfied for this disease by transmission of gastritis to bacteria-free piglets. Marshall's self-experiment was a dramatic event that was reported in the popular press, but it had little impact on the acceptance of the bacterial theory of ulcers.

As of the mid-1990s, Koch's third postulate had not been fulfilled for peptic ulcers. Marshall's self-induced case of gastritis cleared up on its own, so he did not have the continuing infection that might have contributed to an ulcer. In fact, most people who have *H. pylori* infections do not develop get ulcers. John Graham (1995) used the lack of fulfillment of Koch's postulates to cast doubt on the hypothesis that ulcers are caused by bacteria, contending that *H. pylori* is nothing more than an opportunist that accompanies ulcers. He maintained (p. 1096) that "as long as Koch's postulates remain unfulfilled for *H. pylori* as a cause of peptic ulcers or gastric malignancy, it is quite wrong for authoritative medical bodies to attempt to produce consensus documents that suggest that the eradication of *H. pylori* is an essential component of preventive or healing therapy." He thus challenged the National Institutes of Health (NIH) report that recommended such therapy (National Institutes of Health Consensus Development Panel 1994).

If Koch's postulates were indeed a necessary condition of showing that a microorganism causes a disease, then we would have to delay acceptance of the hypothesis that bacteria cause ulcers. However, the history of medical microbiology shows that, although Koch's postulates help provide a convincing demonstration of a causal relation, they are not the only means of establishing causality. Koch himself encountered difficulty in fulfilling the third postulate (transmission of disease) for cholera, which he was convinced was caused by a bacterium even though it did not produce the disease in any other animal. Even today, there are diseases such as typhoid fever and leprosy that cannot be reproduced in experimental animals with features resembling the human illness; nevertheless, their microbial causes have long been recognized (Evans 1993, p. 31). Koch's second postulate (growth in culture) is also not always satisfiable: The microorganisms responsible for leprosy, syphilis, and malaria still elude growth in pure culture. Moreover, the second postulate does not apply to viruses, which cannot be grown in pure culture.

Why is fulfillment of Koch's postulates such an impressive demonstration of causality? Fulfilling the first postulate merely shows correlation between an organism and a disease, and the correlation might be accidental or the result of another causal factor. Fulfilling the second postulate shows that the organism is a clearly identifiable agent that might be responsible for disease. Fulfilling the third postulate is significant, because it involves an experimental manipulation, in which the potential causal agent, the microorganism, has a dramatic effect on the disease: It introduces the disease to a new animal. Koch's third postulate is important, not because it has some special probative status but because it is a vivid kind of manipulation that serves to show the efficacy of a particular cause and to rule out other possible causes (see chapter 7).

Other kinds of manipulation or intervention are possible in medical microbiology. Pasteur demonstrated that the organisms he had isolated from diseases such as rabies could be used in attenuated form to prevent the diseases. Hence, we should count the prevention of a disease by means of attenuated organisms as a manipulation relevant to establishing causality, in addition to the transmission of a disease. A third significant manipulation is cure of the disease by eradication of the organism. This kind of intervention was not available in Koch's day, since antibiotics were only developed in the 1930s and 1940s, but we shall see in the next section that it has played a major role in convincing many medical researchers that bacteria cause ulcers.

TABLE 4.1

Criteria for Causation

1. *Prevalence* of the disease should be significantly higher in those exposed to the putative cause than in matched control subjects not so exposed.
2. *Exposure* to the putative cause should be present more commonly in those with the disease than in control subjects without the disease when all risk factors are held constant.
3. *Incidence* of the disease should be significantly higher in those exposed to the putative cause than in those not so exposed, as shown in prospective studies.
4. *Temporally*, the disease should follow exposure to the putative agent with a distribution of incubation periods on a bell-shaped curve.
5. A *spectrum* of host responses should follow exposure to the putative agent along a logical biological gradient from mild to severe.
6. A *measurable host response* (e.g., antibody, cancer cells) after exposure to the putative cause should *regularly* appear in those lacking this response before exposure or should increase in magnitude if present before exposure; this pattern should not occur in people not so exposed.
7. *Experimental reproduction* of the disease should occur in higher incidence in animals or humans appropriately exposed to the putative cause than in those not so exposed; this exposure may be deliberate in volunteers, experimentally induced in the laboratory, or demonstrated in a controlled regulation of natural exposure.
8. *Elimination or modification* of the putative cause or of the vector carrying it (e.g., via control of polluted water or smoke or removal of the specific agent) should decrease the incidence of the disease.
9. *Prevention* or *modification* of the host's response on exposure to the putative cause (e.g., via immunization, drug to lower cholesterol, specific lymphocyte transfer factor in cancer) should decrease or eliminate the disease.
10. The whole thing should make biological and epidemiological sense.

Source: Adapted from Evans (1993, p. 174).

Since the time of Koch, new technology has made available other kinds of information concerning diseases, such as determining whether antibodies to an agent are produced in people who acquire the disease. According to Evans (1993), Koch's postulates have not been fulfilled for relating Epstein-Barr virus to infectious mononucleosis, since the virus cannot be grown in the laboratory and a susceptible experimental animal has not been found. Evidence has accumulated, however, that antibody to the virus is regularly absent prior to illness and regularly appears during clinical infectious mononucleosis. Table 4.1 shows the ten criteria for causation that Evans (1993) offers for establishing a cause for a disease.

Evan's first criterion, prevalence, is satisfied for peptic ulcers and *H. pylori*, as shown by the original study of Marshall and Warren (1984) and much subsequent research. I am not aware of studies showing that criteria 2 through 6 have been satisfied. Criterion 7, a weaker form of Koch's third postulate, has not been satisfied for peptic ulcers, which have not been experimentally reproduced. But criteria 2 through 7 are meant to provide only various sources of evidence concerning causal relations, not necessary conditions for demonstrating causality. Evan's eighth criterion, that elimination of the putative cause should decrease the incidence of the disease, has been strikingly employed in the case involving bacteria and ulcers. Criterion 9, prevention of the disease, has not yet been satisfied, although work on a vaccine for *H. pylori* is underway. Criterion 10 is a general condition that a causal hypothesis fit with other biological knowledge; its relevance to the case involving ulcers and bacteria is discussed at the end of this chapter.

CAUSATION AND CURE

By far, the most impressive evidence that *H. pylori* causes peptic ulcers is the demonstration that eradication of *H. pylori* strongly contributes to the elimination of ulcers and the prevention of their recurrence. I briefly review the relevant studies and explain how they answer doubts that have been raised about whether the association between ulcers and bacteria is causal rather than mere co–occurrence.

Marshall and Warren (1984, p. 1314), remarking on their study that found a strong correlation between bacterial infection and ulcers, claimed that the correlation was not sufficient to show a cause-and-effect relation. In 1985 and 1986, they collaborated with the microbiologist C. Stewart Goodwin and other researchers on a prospective double-blind trial of duodenal ulcer relapse after eradication of the bacteria. One hundred patients with both duodenal ulcer and *H. pylori* infection were randomly assigned to eight weeks of treatment with either cimetidine or bismuth, and with either the antibiotic tinidazole or a placebo, producing four treatment groups. (The rationale of details of the experiment and the nature of the collaboration it required are discussed in chapters 5 and 6.) The major result was that ulcer healing occurred in ninety-two percent of patients in whom *H. pylori* was not detected at ten weeks, whereas only sixty-one percent of patients with persistent *H. pylori* healed. After twelve months, relapse occurred in eighty-four percent of patients in which *H. pylori* had not been eradicated but in only twenty-one percent of the patients without continuing *H. pylori* infection. Marshall et al. (1988) concluded that the results imply that *H. pylori* is the most important etiological factor so far described for duodenal ulcer. A seven-year follow-up examination found that an active ulcer remained in twenty percent of *H. pylori*–positive patients but in only three percent of *H. pylori*–negative patients (Forbes et al. 1994). Similar results have been reported by Coghlan et al. (1987) and by Rauws and Tytgat (1990).

Between 1988 and 1990, David Graham and his colleagues in Houston compared patients (with ulcers and *H. pylori* infection) receiving (1) ranitidine versus (2) ranitidine plus triple therapy, consisting of bismuth and two antibiotics, tetracycline and metronidazole. After two years, they found that continuing infection with *H. pylori* was a strong predictor of ulcer recurrence (D. Y. Graham et al. 1992). All forty-seven patients whose ulcers healed while receiving ranitidine still had *H. pylori* infection at the end of therapy, and ninety-five percent of them re-developed ulcers. In contrast, none of the patients in whom *H. pylori* was eradicated became reinfected. The effect was almost as strong for gastric ulcer as for peptic ulcer. Graham confidently editorialized that *H. pylori* infection is the most common known cause of peptic ulcer and accounts for the majority of cases, and that *H. pylori* ulcer disease can be cured (D. Y. Graham 1993; D. Y. Graham and Go 1993).

Critics of the bacterial theory of ulcers argued that the provision of bismuth might be the cause of ulcer healing in such experiments, rather than the eradication of the bacteria (Peterson 1991). Bismuth causes patients to produce dark stools, so the patients were not really blind to which treatment they had received; further, bismuth might have an effect on the mucous layer that is more important than bismuth's known antibacterial properties. But Austrian researchers found that giving amoxicillin and metronidazole without bismuth was also a successful treatment for duodenal ulcer, which recurred in eighty-five percent of patients given only ranitidine but in only 2 percent of patients given ranitidine and antibiotics (Hentschel et al. 1993). Dutch researchers conducted a study to determine how important acid inhibition was to the eradication of ulcers, and they found that triple therapy with bismuth, tetracycline, and metronadizole alone provided an eighty-three percent cure rate, compared with ninety-eight percent with the addition of the acid inhibitor omeprazole (de Boer et al. 1995). Thus, the acid inhibitor clearly helps, but the antibiotic treatment alone is highly effective for curing ulcers (Hosking et al. 1994). Antibacterial drugs, not just bismuth and antacids, play a key role in curing ulcers.

The NIH regularly convenes consensus development conferences to make recommendations concerning medical treatments. The conference that met in February 1994 produced a consensus document advising that ulcer patients with *H. pylori* infection be treated with antibiotics. The document stated that "the strongest evidence for the pathogenic role of *H. pylori* in peptic ulcer disease is the marked decrease in recurrence rate of ulcers following the eradication of infection. The prevention of recurrence following *H. pylori* eradication is less well documented for gastric ulcer than for duodenal ulcer, but the available data suggest similar efficacy" (National Institutes of Health Consensus Development Panel 1994, p. 66). Medical discussion has clearly shifted away from whether bacteria cause ulcers to methods for best treating the bacteria that cause ulcers. Correlational studies have also suggested that *H. pylori* is a causal agent in the development of gastric cancer and coronary heart disease, although these hypotheses have not yet been supported by studies that produce cures. (See chapters 6 and 12 for further discussion of medical consensus panels.)

The causal role of *H. pylori* in peptic ulcers thus seems to have been established without satisfying Koch's third postulate. Manipulation involving the transmission of disease is only one kind of evidence for causality. Acceptance of the hypothesis that peptic ulcers are caused by *H. pylori* depends on assessing various kinds of evidence in the context of alternative hypotheses. The next section lays out the evidential structure now supporting the bacterial theory of ulcers.

An important philosophical question remains: What does it mean to say that bacteria cause ulcers? A Humean regularity theory of causality would interpret this question as a claim that the bacteria and ulcers are universally associated, but this is clearly not the case. Many people with *H. pylori* infection do not develop peptic ulcers, and some cases of peptic ulcers occur because of the use of nonsteroidal anti-inflammatory drugs such as aspirin and ibuprofen. Approximately thirty percent of gastric ulcers are thought to be related to these medications. A probabilistic theory of causality would note that the probability of ulcers given the presence *H. pylori* infection is much higher than the probability of ulcers otherwise. This conclusion is true but irrelevant if the increased probability is accidental or the result of a common cause that encourages both ulcers and bacteria. Medical researchers want to know *why* the probability of getting ulcers is so much greater in people with *H. pylori* infection. To answer this question, they are now investigating causal mechanisms such as one proposed by D. Y. Graham (1991b) in Figure 4.1. It now appears that *H. pylori* infection increases acid secretion. Figure 4.1 suggests a series of processes by which infection can lead to gastrin release, acid secretion, and eventually to an ulcer. Research is underway to fill in the gaps about these processes (Olbe et al. 1996) as well as to learn about the more fundamental genetic and biochemical mechanisms that enable *H. pylori* to colonize the stomach. The complete genome for *H. pylori* has now been deciphered, and the protein that allows the bacteria to attach to stomach cells has been identified. The statement that bacteria cause ulcers is thus not a comment about regularities or probabilities, but it is rather an assertion that there is a continuous process connecting infection and the development of ulcers (cf. Salmon 1984; Schaffner 1993). The nature of medical causality is discussed more generally in chapter 7.

REJECTION, ACCEPTANCE, AND EXPLANATORY COHERENCE

Evans's tenth criterion for causality requires that a causal hypothesis make biological and epidemiological sense: The hypothesis must fit with other beliefs about how organisms function and how diseases develop. Other epidemi-

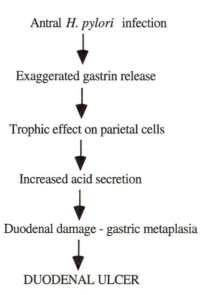

Antral *H. pylori* infection

Exaggerated gastrin release

Trophic effect on parietal cells

Increased acid secretion

Duodenal damage - gastric metaplasia

DUODENAL ULCER

Figure 4.1 The role of *Helicobacter pylori* infection in the pathogenesis of exaggerated gastrin release and its theoretical role in patients with duodenal ulcer. Adapted from D. Y. Graham (1991b), p. 307. Graham elsewhere indicates that the causality is still more complicated, involving environmental factors, genetic predispositions, and the possible interaction of acid secretion and bacterial infection. See Figure 7.2.

ologists, Susser (1973) and Elwood (1988), similarly specify *coherence* with what is known about the disease, with the possible cause considered a factor relevant to assessing causality. Many epistemologists, for example, BonJour (1985), Harman (1986), and Lehrer (1990), have taken coherence to be the basis for all knowledge claims, but they have remained vague about what constitutes coherence and how it can be assessed. In contrast, Thagard and Verbeurgt (1998) have offered a characterization of coherence sufficiently precise that algorithms for computing it are available. This view of coherence can be used to explain why the hypothesis that bacteria cause ulcers was widely rejected when first proposed in 1983, and also to explain why it was widely accepted by 1995.

The most powerful alternative to a coherentist explanation is Bayesian: One could say that the hypothesis that bacteria cause ulcers was improbable given the evidence in 1983 but probable given the evidence in 1995. To work this out in sufficient detail to apply Bayes's theorem, one would need to specify numerous probabilities, such as the prior probability of the hypothesis that bacteria cause ulcers, the probability of each piece of evidence given that hypothesis, and the probability of each piece of evidence. I know of no way of arriving at non-arbitrary values for such probabilities, nor of any plausible interpretation of the meaning of such probabilities, which obviously differ from the frequencies of occurrences of events in populations. Moreover, because the aim in this series of chapters is to provide a naturalistic explanation of scientific developments, the explanation of belief change must be psychologically plausible. There is abundant evidence that human psychology often deviates from the canons of probabilistic reasoning (Kahneman et al. 1982). Hence, I pursue a much simpler and more psychologically plausible line of explanation based on coherence.

The kind of coherence most relevant to the evaluation of the hypothesis that ulcers are caused by bacteria is *explanatory* coherence. Thagard (1992b) provides a set of principles for establishing coherence relations among hypotheses and evidence. For the case involving ulcers and bacteria, the most relevant principle is that when a hypothesis explains evidence or another hypothesis, the two propositions cohere with each other such that there is a positive constraint between them, encouraging that they both be either accepted or rejected. On the other hand, if two hypotheses contradict each other, or if they offer competing explanations of some piece of evidence, then they are incoherent with each other; this result should lead to the acceptance of one and the rejection of the other. Pieces of evidence are given priority, not in the sense that they must be accepted but in the sense that there is a constraint that will encourage their acceptance. This constraint can be modeled by supposing that there is a special element—evidence—which is accepted and coheres with all the pieces of evidence.

Let us now see why the hypothesis that ulcers cause bacteria was not coherent with most researchers' beliefs in 1984 but was coherent for many researchers in 1995. Figure 4.2 provides a rough sketch of the positive and negative constraints on the various beliefs of a typical gastroenterologist in 1983. It shows that this hypothesis was problematic for at least two reasons. First, it competed with the well-established hypothesis that peptic ulcers are caused by excess acidity. The most impressive evidence for this hypothesis was the healing of ulcers using drugs such as cimetidine. Second, the hypothesis that gastric bacteria exist was incompatible with the accepted assumption that the stomach was too acidic for permanent bacterial growth. Because only a few researchers had observed the bacteria and there was only a small amount of evidence connecting ulcers and bacteria, it is not surprising that Marshall's hypothesis was greeted with incredulity. The bacteria that Warren observed could be explained as the result of contamination. Maximizing coherence— that is, accepting and rejecting propositions in a way that maximizes the satisfaction of constraints—required rejecting the hypothesis that ulcers are caused by bacteria.

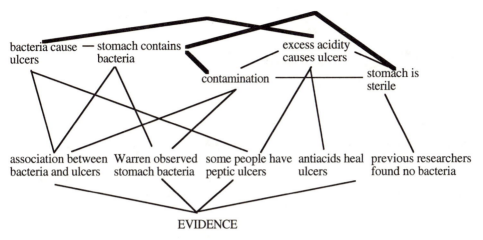

Figure 4.2. Coherence relations in assessing the acceptability of the hypothesis in 1983 that bacteria cause ulcers. Thin lines indicate positive constraints based on hypotheses explaining evidence, and thick lines indicate negative constraints based on contradiction or competition.

Although Figure 4.2 reflects the belief systems of many gastroenterologists in 1983, the belief systems of Warren and Marshall were quite different. Warren's systematic observations made it clear to himself and Marshall that the stomach does contain gastric spiral bacteria and hence is not sterile; they knew that contamination was not a plausible explanation of Warren's results. Marshall was relatively new to gastroenterology but had a background in infectious diseases, so a bacteriological explanation of ulcers was less alien to him than to most gastroenterologists. But in 1983, their beliefs were at odds with accepted wisdom, and controlled studies to demonstrate a causal link between bacteria and ulcers had not been conducted.

By 1995, the picture had changed considerably. By then, countless researchers had studied *H. pylori*, so the view of the stomach as bacteria free had dropped out altogether. More than half a dozen studies from different researchers using different techniques had shown that ulcers can be cured using antibiotics that eradicate the bacteria. In addition, some researchers had conjectured that *H. pylori* increases acidity and that eradication of *H. pylori* decreases acidity. Figure 4.3 shows part of the coherence network involving the hypotheses being considered in 1995. Maximizing coherence therefore requires acceptance of the hypothesis that ulcers are caused by bacteria. More constraints are satisfied if the hypothesis that bacteria cause ulcers is included in the set of accepted elements than if it is included in the set of rejected elements.

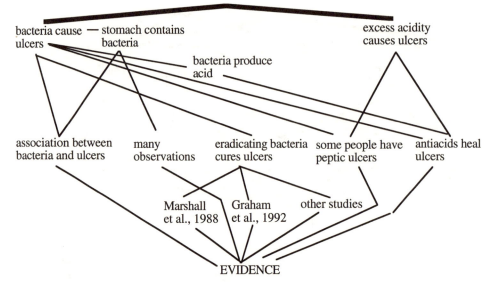

bacteria cause — stomach contains
ulcers ————— bacteria

excess acidity
causes ulcers

bacteria produce
acid

association between
bacteria and ulcers

many
observations

eradicating bacteria
cures ulcers

some people have
peptic ulcers

antiacids heal
ulcers

Marshall
et al., 1988

Graham
et al., 1992

other studies

EVIDENCE

Figure 4.3. Coherence relations in assessing the acceptability of the hypothesis in 1995 that bacteria cause ulcers. Thin lines indicate positive constraints based on hypotheses explaining evidence, and thick lines indicate negative constraints based on contradiction or competition.

Computer simulations using my explanatory coherence program ECHO show that maximizing coherence (given the relations in Figure 4.2) leads one to reject the hypothesis that bacteria cause ulcers, whereas maximizing coherence (given the relations in Figure 4.3) leads one to accept the hypothesis. Similar simulations have been used to model belief change in many scientific revolutions (Nowak and Thagard 1992a, 1992b; Thagard 1992b). Eliasmith and Thagard (1997) argue that the acceptance of the wave theory of light is much better understood in coherence terms than in probabilistic terms. In contrast to probabilistic reasoning, coherence assessment is computationally efficient (Thagard in press).

If explanatory coherence now requires accepting the bacterial theory of ulcers, why are a few medical researchers still skeptical and why are some physicians still not treating ulcers with antibiotics? One reason is that communication is slow: The relevant research has appeared in medical journals only during the past few years, and practitioners have much to do besides reading medical journals. Another reason is that explanatory coherence is not the only kind involved in medical decisions, which are practical as well as theoretical. Treatment of peptic ulcers with cimetidine and ranitidine is a tried-and-true way of making most ulcer patients feel better. Triple therapy with antibiotics and bismuth requires as many as fifteen pills a day and can produce nausea and diarrhea. Conservatism in adopting new treatments is not necessarily a bad trait in a medical practitioner, since novel therapies may have unforeseen side effects. Chapter 12 describes current attempts by medical organizations to make antibiotic treatment of ulcers more widespread.

For a naturalistic explanation of belief change, the coherence account must be psychologically plausible. There is indirect evidence that it is plausible: Parallel constraint satisfaction models using connectionist algorithms have been widely applied, in recent work in cognitive science, to psychological phenomena that include word recognition, vision and imagery, analogy, language comprehension, and social impression formation (Holyoak and Spellman 1993; Holyoak and Thagard 1995; Kunda and Thagard 1996; Read and Marcus-Newhall 1993; Schank and Ranney 1992). Moreover, the explanatory coherence model ECHO has been used to account for the results of various psychological experiments. It is therefore plausible that the belief change experienced by many medical researchers and practitioners concerning the cause of ulcers was produced by a process of assessing explanatory coherence. The Cognitive Explanation Schema for belief acquisition in chapter 1 can accordingly be specified as follows:

Coherence Explanation Schema
   Explanation target:
   Why did a **scientist** accept a **hypothesis**?
   Explanatory pattern:
   The **scientist** had **mental representations** of hypotheses and evidence linked by explanation relations.
   The **scientist** had **mental procedures** for evaluating the coherence of the various hypotheses and evidence.
   The **scientist's** coherence evaluation produced the acceptance of the **hypothesis**.

When scientists maximize coherence while taking into account all relevant evidence and hypotheses, their inferences are rational, in that they meet the highest reasoning standards compatible with people's cognitive abilities.

CONCLUSION

Initially, Marshall thought that his hypothesis about a bacterial cause for ulcers would gain quick acceptance. Discouraged by the negative reception, he came to believe that only the development of a new generation of gastroenterologists would bring acceptance of the new ideas. This prediction has proved to be unduly pessimistic, even as the early estimate of quick acceptance was unduly optimistic. Increasingly, the view that peptic ulcers are caused by *H. pylori* is being accepted by medical researchers, although acceptance by practitioners has been slower. Not surprisingly, the process has been complex, and a variety of studies have contributed to displaying the greater explanatory coherence of the new theory.

I have shown how the hypothesis that *H. pylori* is the principal cause of peptic ulcers—which was largely rejected as absurd in 1983—could be on its way to medical orthodoxy in 1995. Satisfying Koch's postulates is not a necessary condition of showing that a microorganism causes a disease. Curing the disease by eliminating the microorganism is a powerful manipulation that provides substantial evidence that the microorganism causes the disease, and this kind of intervention has been repeatedly successful in the case presented here. However, accepting the hypothesis that bacteria cause ulcers is not just a matter of appreciating one kind of evidence but rather of appreciating how the hypothesis coheres with various kinds of evidence and with other hypotheses. For most researchers, the claim that ulcers cause bacteria was not part of the most coherent account in 1983, but it was maximally coherent for well-informed scientists by 1995.

Cognitive coherence is, however, only part of the story about why the bacterial theory of ulcers has been increasingly accepted. This chapter has treated belief change as a largely psychological phenomenon, a process in the minds of medical researchers. But the development of medical science also requires attention to researchers' interactions with the world by means of instruments and experiments and attention to researchers' social interactions with each other and with other parts of society. A full naturalistic account of the rise of the bacterial theory of ulcers should eventually specify how the cognitive aspects of belief formation and change described in this paper interact with the physical and social aspects of the development of science (see chapters 5 and 6).

SUMMARY

Between 1983 and 1995, the reaction to the hypothesis that bacteria cause peptic ulcers changed from strong skepticism to widespread acceptance. One early problem in this process was that the hypothesis did not satisfy Koch's postulates, which require that a disease be induced experimentally by an organism claimed to cause the disease. However, Koch's postulates are only one way of establishing causality, and the experiments showing that eradication of *H. pylori* usually cures ulcers provided another effective way. In 1983, the hypothesis that bacteria cause ulcers was not coherent with accepted beliefs, but by 1995, the hypothesis had acquired considerable explanatory coherence with the evidence and with other beliefs.

CHAPTER 5

Ulcers and Bacteria:
Instruments and Experiments

My DESCRIPTION of the cognitive processes involved in the discovery, development, and acceptance of the bacterial theory of ulcers might have left the impression that science is all in the mind. But only part of the story of the bacterial theory of ulcers is psychological. This chapter discusses the important role of physical interaction with the world by means of instruments and experiments. The main questions I address are the following:

1. What instruments contributed to the development and acceptance of the new theory?

2. What kinds of experiments contributed to the development and acceptance of the new theory?

3. How did theorizing and experimentation interact in the development of new experiments and hypotheses?

INSTRUMENTS

Both the discovery and the evaluation of the bacterial theory of ulcers would have been impossible without several kinds of scientific instruments that make possible the examination of bacteria and the gastrointestinal system. Microscopes, endoscopes, and other technologies played crucial roles in investigations concerning *Helicobacter pylori* and ulcers.

Microscopes

Because bacteria are very small, typically ½ to 5 microns, they cannot be observed by the naked eye. Around the year 1600, spectacle makers in the Netherlands discovered how to produce and combine lenses to increase magnification of small objects. In approximately 1673, a Dutch draper, Antony van Leeuwenhoek, became interested in the new devices for magnification. He began building his own single-lens microscopes, achieving magnifying power as high as 275× with resolving power approaching one micron (Bradbury 1968). Leeuwenhoek described his observations in letters to the Royal Society of London and in 1676 reported finding "little animals" in water (Dobell 1958, p. 133). These bacteria were much smaller than the protozoa that he had previously observed, but their medical significance was not appreciated until the work of Pasteur in the mid-nineteenth century.

Gastric spiral bacteria were microscopically observed as early as the 1890s, and in the 1970s Steer and Colin-Jones (1975) reported the co–occurrence of gastric bacteria and ulceration. Steer and Colin-Jones were unsuccessful, however, in attempts to culture the bacteria, which they identified as *Pseudomonas aeruginosa*. In 1979, Robin Warren was using an Orthoplan optical microscope at 250× magnification to examine histological sections from patients with gastritis. He noticed the unexpected presence of spiral bacteria and then used an oil immersion microscope capable of 1,000× magnification to examine them more closely. To observe the morphology of the bacteria more clearly, he requested a Warthin-Starry silver stain on gastric biopsies and was able to see many spiral organisms. He had previously used this kind of stain for observing the spirochetes that are responsible for syphilis. Staining of bacteria, which originated with Herman Hoffman in 1869, makes possible much clearer observation of their structure (Bulloch 1979).

All subsequent experiments observing the correlation of the bacteria and various diseases—as well as experiments finding that eradicating the bacteria can cure diseases such as gastritis and ulcers—used microscopes to determine the presence or absence of bacteria in the gastric biopsies. Without microscopes, bacteria would never have been discovered, and the bacterial theory of ulcers would never have been developed and accepted.

Although most of the clinical research involving *H. pylori* has been performed using optical microscopes, electron microscopes proved very useful in identifying the detailed morphology of the newly discovered species of bacteria. In 1982, just after the first cultures of *H. pylori* were produced, Barry Marshall delivered specimens to an electron microscopist, John Armstrong, who produced the first electron micrographs of the bacteria (Marshall 1989). Armstrong identified the essential morphological features—four or five sheathed flagella—that differentiated the gastric spiral bacteria from the species *Campylobacter jejuni*. Subsequent investigations, using electron microscopes and other technologies such as RNA sequencing, provided evidence that the bacteria did not belong in the genus *Campylobacter* and led to the naming of a new genus, *Helicobacter* (Goodwin and Worsley 1993). Without these instruments, which permitted much more detailed observation of the structure and properties of the gastric bacteria, the conceptual change that produced a reclassification of the bacteria would not have been possible. Figure 5.1 is a photograph of *H. pylori*.

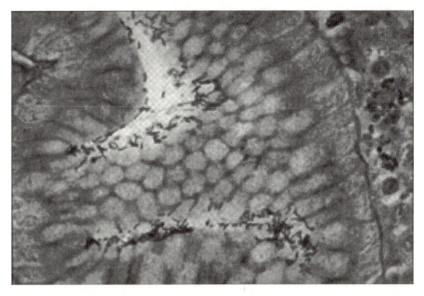

Figure 5.1. Microscopic photograph of *Helicobacter pylori*, used by permission of Joel K. Greenson, MD. For a color version, see http://www.pds.med.umich.edu/users/greenson/HP-SILVER.GIF.

Endoscopes

Production of the gastric biopsy slides that investigators examine microscopically employs an instrument that came into general use only in the 1960s: the fiber optic endoscope. Endoscopes, such as gastroscopes, proctoscopes, and esophagoscopes, are tubular instruments used to examine the inside of body cavities. After unsuccessful nineteenth-century experiments with candles and incandescent lamps as light sources, the first usable straight gastroscope was produced in 1911 (Hirschowitz 1993). But the available instruments were difficult to use and often did not allow adequate inspection of the stomach. A semiflexible gastroscope produced in 1932 was still uncomfortable for patients and could be used to examine only limited portions of the stomach. Endoscopy was rarely used for diagnosis of upper gastrointestinal tract diseases, which depended instead on barium x-rays.

In the 1950s, a new technology for the transmission of information became available. Hopkins and Kapany (1954) designed a flexible fiberscope that used glass fibers encased in a cladding to direct light along a curved path. Fiber optics have since become the main medium for carrying all types of telecommunications, but one of their first applications was the manufacture of endoscopes for medical exploration. In 1957, Basil Hirschowitz and his colleagues produced the first fiber-optic gastroscope, and such instruments were in clinical use by the early 1960s. Improved instruments included biopsy channels for taking tissue samples from the stomach and, after 1983, video screens on which the endoscopist and others could observe the stomach.

By the 1970s, endoscopy had become a standard technique for gastroenterologists, who, by inserting a tube with fiber optics down the throat of patient, could view the inside of the stomach. Using this technology, an ulcer is immediately visible as a sore or hole in the lining of the stomach (gastric ulcer) or as a sore on the upper part of the intestine (duodenal ulcer). Endoscopy not only makes possible identification of ulcers but also enables gastroenterologists to take samples of stomach tissue by means of a miniature pincer attached to the end of the endoscope. They can therefore submit tissue samples to pathologists for further examinations. Warren's observations of bacteria in stomach tissue in the late 1970s were made on samples obtained via endoscopy. On the World Wide Web, the Atlas of Gastrointestinal Endoscopy contains a picture of a modern fiber-optic endoscope as well as graphic photographs of stomach ulcers (available at http://www.mindspring.com/dmmmd/atlas_1.html).

Endoscopy has played a crucial role in the experiments that have contributed to the acceptance of the bacterial theory of ulcers. Definitive diagnosis of a peptic ulcer is made by endoscopic observation of lesions, and samples gained through endoscopy are crucial for determining the presence or absence of *H. pylori*. The early experiments that found a correlation between the presence of bacteria and ulcers (described later) and the later, more conclusive experiments demonstrating that antibiotics can eradicate bacteria and cure ulcers, all depended on internal examination and tissue sampling using endoscopes. Without endoscopy to provide stomach samples, the bacterial theory of ulcers would never have been discovered or validated.

Originally, the only way to diagnose *H. pylori* infection was by endoscopic biopsy of the gastric mucosa. But Graham and his colleagues designed a non-invasive detection method based on the fact that *H. pylori* produces large amounts of urease that buffers it from gastric acid (D. Y. Graham et al. 1987; see also Marshall et al. 1991). Using this technique, patients suspected of having *H. pylori* in their stomachs are given a small quantity of urea containing an isotope of carbon. If urease is present, it reacts with the urea to form carbon dioxide containing the isotope, which is detected by having the patient breathe into a balloon. Patients with stomach distress can be diagnosed regarding *H. pylori* infection without undergoing the expensive and somewhat unpleasant experience of endoscopy and, if necessary, immediately treated with antibiotics. Cutler et al. (1995) reported that urea breath tests are as effective as endoscopic biopsy for diagnosing infection. Urea breath tests did not contribute to the discovery or validation of the bacterial theory of ulcers, but they promise to be of increasing importance in the future treatment of gastritis and ulcers. For details on how the urea breath test works, see the World Wide

Web page of Barry Marshall's *Helicobacter* Foundation (available at http://www.helico.com/).

Significance of Scientific Instruments

The centrality of the use of microscopes, endoscopes, and other instruments makes it clear that gastroenterologists and microbiologists are not disembodied researchers spinning ideas in their heads, removed from contact with the world. Although their use of instruments is guided by their conceptual systems, those systems do not determine the observations that researchers make through instrumental interventions with microorganisms and bodily tissues. Scientific change derives from technology as well as from psychology. Formation of the initial mental representation of *gastric spiral bacteria* and refinement of the concept into *Campylobacter pyloridis* and finally *H. pylori* required physical processes by which researchers took stomach samples using endoscopes and observed the extracted bacteria using optical and electron microscopes (see the discussion of reference in chapter 10). These physical processes are much more complex than simple sensory observation, since substantial skill and training are required to obtain and interpret the results of endoscopy and microscopy. Nevertheless, the physical processes of instrument use and the mental processes of interpretation of data provided by the instruments yield substantial agreement across time and across researchers. Agreement, however, arises not merely because of the isolated use of instruments but also because of the systematic conducting of medical experiments.

EXPERIMENTS

Recent philosophy and history of science has paid increasing attention to the role of experimentation in scientific research (see, for example, Ackermann 1985, Galison 1987, Gooding 1990, and Hacking 1983). Attention to experimentation has valuably redressed an imbalance toward theory in previous science studies, but almost all the investigations have concerned experiments in physics. Medical experimentation takes on quite different forms, which I now describe with particular reference to the experiments that were important to the development and acceptance of the bacterial theory of ulcers.

Medical Experiments

Hennekens and Buring (1987) describe six kinds of studies that can be used to investigate the distributions and causes of diseases.

1. *Correlational studies* use data from entire populations to compare disease frequencies between different groups during the same period of time or in the same population at different points of time. For example, there is a positive correlation across countries between the consumption of large amounts of meat and the incidence of colon cancer. Such correlational studies can be a useful source of hypotheses about the causes of diseases, but they are weak for evaluating causal claims because of the unknown effects of other variables.

2. *Case reports and case studies* consist of detailed descriptions of one or more patients with a particular disease. For example, the occurrence of a particular kind of pneumonia in five young, previously healthy young men in Los Angeles in 1980 suggested the existence of a previously unknown disease (AIDS) and led to the conjecture that the cause of the disease might be related to sexual behavior.

3. *Cross-sectional surveys* are large studies that collect extensive information from individuals at a particular point in time. They make possible calculation of the frequencies of various diseases in relation to age, sex, race, socioeconomic variables, medication use, cigarette smoking, and other risk factors. Although such studies can be suggestive about the causes of disease, they are never definitive, since causes and effects are difficult to disentangle. When individuals with cancer are found to have lower levels of serum beta-carotene, for example, it is not clear whether the lower levels are a cause or an effect of the cancer.

Hennekens and Buring (1987) contrast these three kinds of *descriptive* study with *analytic* studies, in which an investigator assembles groups of individuals to make an explicit comparison of the risk of disease between those exposed to a factor and those not exposed.

4. *Case-control studies* select a group of patients who have a disease and compare them with a control group of patients who do not have the disease. For example, a group of patients who have a particular kind of cancer can be compared with a group of similar patients who do not have cancer. The comparison can examine various potentially relevant variables such as diet, smoking, medication use, and so on.

5. *Cohort studies* differ from case-control studies temporally: Subjects are classified based on the presence or absence of exposure to a factor and are then followed over time to determine the comparative development of disease in each exposure group. In the early 1950s, for example, the Framingham Heart Study established a cohort of more than five thousand people identified with respect to medical history, cigarette smoking, and a variety of laboratory variables. Reexamination of members of the cohort at regular intervals has identified numerous risk factors for cardiovascular disease.

6. *Intervention studies* (clinical trials) are a special kind of cohort study in which the exposure status of the individuals is randomly determined by the investigator. The advantage of random assignment to exposure and nonexposure conditions is that it controls for the effects of other risk factors, both recognized and unrecognized. For example, randomly assigning patients with hypertension into groups that receive or do not receive a medication can provide evidence of the effectiveness of the medication. Hennekens and Buring (1987, pp. 26–27) remark that "when well designed and conducted, intervention studies can indeed provide the most direct epidemiologic evidence on which to judge whether an exposure causes or prevents a disease."

Ulcers and Bacteria: Case Studies

Experimental work on ulcers and bacteria has moved through increasing stages of sophistication, from case studies to a cross-sectional survey to intervention studies. Warren's observation noticing of an association between spiral bacteria and gastritis was based on 135 gastric biopsy specimens collected between 1979 and 1982 (Warren and Marshall 1983). In July 1981, Warren gave Marshall a list of 25 patients in whom large numbers of gastric spiral bacteria were present, but Marshall's examination of the patients' case notes did not reveal any characteristic clinical features (Marshall 1989). In September 1981, Marshall used the antibiotic tetracycline to treat a patient with abdominal pain of unknown origin, and the patient's symptom and gastritis were completely resolved. Marshall and Warren then began a more systematic investigation of the clinical significance of the bacteria.

The 1982 Cross-Sectional Study

Between April and June of 1982, Marshall and his colleagues collected biopsy specimens from one hundred patients who had been scheduled for endoscopy. Warren received the biopsies and examined them for the presence of the bacteria. Marshall coded the endoscopy reports for the one hundred patients to record the occurrences of gastritis and gastric and duodenal ulcers. Questionnaires, endoscopy reports, and microbiology results were coded independently in separate departments, and the complete results for individual patients were not known until the statistician had received all the data (Marshall and Warren 1984). In October 1982, Marshall received printouts from the statistician and immediately noticed a strong association between gastritis and the presence of gastric spiral bacteria (Marshall 1989). Only later did he notice that all thirteen patients with duodenal ulcer also had the organism. When Marshall and Warren (1984) reported these associations in *Lancet*, they conjectured that the bacteria were causally related to gastritis and probably also to peptic ulceration. Intervention studies were needed before stronger claims about causal relations could be made convincingly. Marshall et al. (1985) reported a replication at Fremantle Hospital of the results of the 1982 study: that bacterial infection strongly correlated with both gastritis and gastric ulcer. They also reported on the basis of in vitro studies that the bacteria were sensitive to numerous antibiotics, including penicillin, erythromycin, and tetracycline. This sensitivity made possible the cure-based intervention studies described in the next section.

The purpose of the 1982 experiment was not just to determine the medical significance of the bacteria but also to learn more about the nature of the bacteria. From each patient, two biopsy specimens were taken, one which was sent for microscopic examination to Warren, the other which was transported in nutrient broth to the microbiology lab. After many tries, the organism was cultured for the first time in April 1982. Sections were also sent to John Armstrong, the electron microscopist at Perth General Hospital, for ultrastructural examination. Thus, the 1982 experiment involved all the major technologies describe in the last section: optical microscopy, light microscopy, and endoscopy. The experiment also required the various technologies developed in the nineteenth century for culturing and observing bacteria, such as growth media, incubators, and stains.

Intervention: Infection and Cure

As Marshall and Warren (1984) explicitly noted, the 1982 experiment was not sufficient to establish a causal relation between the gastric spiral bacteria and gastric diseases. To establish causality, two kinds of intervention studies were relevant: (1) determining whether people who were given the bacteria developed gastritis or ulcers and (2) eliminating the bacteria in people with gastritis or ulcers to see if doing so eliminates the diseases. Obviously, it would be ethically objectionable to conduct the first kind of study, but in 1984, Marshall performed the experiment on himself, as described in chapter 4. Ten days after Marshall swallowed a culture of the bacteria, gastroscopy and microscopy demonstrated that spiral bacteria had established themselves in Marshall's stomach. On the fourteenth day, Marshall began taking the antibiotic tinidazole, and his symptoms resolved within twenty-four hours. Marshall et al. (1985) described this experiment as an "attempt to fulfil Koch's postulates for pyloric campylobacter" for gastritis. It is standard in medical microbiology to show that a microbe causes a disease by isolating the microbe from an infected animal and transferring it to a new animal that contracts the disease (chapter 4). Because early attempts to cause gastric disease in nonhuman animals using

H. pylori had failed, Marshall's self-experiment was an important part of the evidence that the bacteria cause gastritis. It did not, however, address the question of whether the bacteria cause gastric ulcers, since Marshall was cured before an ulcer could develop.

Between April 1985 and August, 1987, Marshall and numerous colleagues at the Royal Perth Hospital examined one hundred consecutive patients with both duodenal ulcer and *H. pylori* infection to see whether eradication of the bacteria affected ulcer healing or relapse (Marshall et al. 1988). This experiment was double-blind, in that histology and microbiology findings were concealed from both the patients and the physicians managing them. Patients were randomly assigned to receive either the antacid cimetidine or colloidal bismuth subcitrate and either tinidazole or a placebo. The four treatment groups were thus cimetidine + tinidazole, cimetidine + placebo, bismuth + tinidazole, and bismuth + placebo. Bismuth + tinidazole was by far the most effective combination, clearing the infection in twenty of twenty-seven patients. After ten weeks, patients underwent endoscopy. Healing of ulcers had taken place in 92% of patients in whom *H. pylori* bacteria were not detected, compared with only 61% of patients with persistent *H. pylori*. Marshall et al. (1988, p. 1441) concluded: "Our results imply that *C pylori* [*H. pylori*] is the most important aetiologic factor so far described for duodenal ulcer." Many other researchers have conducted similar experiments that show that various kinds of antibiotic therapy are effective at healing both duodenal and gastric ulcers and at preventing their recurrence (chapter 4). The accumulated evidence provided by these intervention studies is such that in 1995 Marshall was awarded the highly prestigious Albert Lasker clinical medical research award "for the visionary discovery that *Helicobacter pylori* causes peptic ulcer disease." I note again that endoscopes and microscopes were essential ingredients in these intervention experiments. The paper by Marshall et al. (1988) has nine authors; see chapter 6 for details of the nature of the collaboration among members of several different medical specialties.

Pilot Experiments

I have summarized the early experiments whose results Marshall and Warren reported in publications. However, looking only at published reports ignores the importance of small pilot experiments that scientists use to determine if they are on the right track before investing more resources in larger studies. Before Marshall and Warren conducted the 1982 study involving one hundred patients, they conducted a smaller preliminary study of twenty patients who underwent endoscopy. Similarly, in 1983, before beginning a major study on the effects of *H. pylori* eradication on ulceration, Marshall carried out a pilot study in which he found that ulcer patients treated with bismuth had a substantially lower relapse rate than did those treated with cimetidine (Taga-met). This study provided early support for the hypothesis that bismuth kills bacteria, thereby healing gastritis and preventing ulcer relapse. Pilot studies are not probative in themselves, but they do play an important role in determining what large-scale experiments are deemed worth performing.

EXPERIMENT AND THEORY

The experimental developments concerning ulcers and bacteria belie several simplistic pictures of how science works. Experimentation and theory interact in ways more complex than any of the following caricatures describes:

1. Inductivist: Scientists conduct experiments to collect data and then generalize the results. Good hypotheses and theories are derived from experimental results.

2. Hypothetico-deductivist: Scientists start with hypotheses and then conduct experiments to test them. If the experiments have the predicted results, the hypotheses are confirmed; otherwise, the hypotheses are refuted.

3. Social constructivist: Experiments are part of the social construction of scientific facts.

The inductivist picture fits best with Marshall and Warren's 1982 experiment, in which they sought to find out whether gastric symptoms and diseases correlate with the occurrence of gastric spiral bacteria. This experiment was not designed to test any specific hypothesis about the medical role of *H. pylori*, but the experiment did not operate in a theoretical vacuum either: Marshall did not know what diseases the bacteria might be associated with, but he did suspect, presumably by analogy with the disease-causing effects of other kinds of bacteria, that *H. pylori* might be the cause of some diseases. The design of the 1982 experiment specifically looked for associations between the presence of the bacteria and the presence of specific diseases of interest: gastritis, gastric ulcer, duodenal ulcer, and other stomach abnormalities. Marshall and Warren were neither simple-minded empiricists, merely collecting experimental data, nor were they theory-blinded deductivists trying to confirm their own predictions. At this stage of the investigation, they had no clear predictions to test.

In contrast, the hypothetic-deductivist picture fits better with the intervention studies that were indeed designed to test the hypotheses that *H. pylori* causes peptic ulcers and that ulcers can be cured by eradicating the bacteria with antibiotics. The logic of the experiment that Marshall et al. reported in 1988 was as follows: If *H. pylori* causes ulcers, then antibiotic treatment of people with ulcers and *H. pylori* infection should cure the ulcers. The experimental design, however, made matters much more complex than this simple conditional allows. The antibiotic tinidazole did not by itself cure ulcers, because the bacteria quickly became resistant to it. The combination treatment of tinidazole + bismuth was much more effective, as Marshall and his colleagues generalized from this study. Hence, they were being simultaneously hypothetic-deductivist and inductivist, using experiments to test hypotheses and also deriving new hypotheses by generalizing from new experimental findings.

MEDICAL REALISM

By the term *medical realism*, I mean that diseases and their causes are real and that scientific investigation can gain knowledge of them. Medical realism is a species of scientific realism, which has been challenged from several directions, including empiricism, conceptualism, and social constructivism. Strict empiricists contend that scientific claims to truth should be restricted to observable phenomena (van Fraassen 1980). Hence, claims that bacteria exist in the stomach, for example, or that bacteria cause ulcers cannot be accepted as true but at best as empirically adequate. Conceptualists conclude from the dramatic kinds of conceptual change that have taken place in the history of science that there is no legitimacy in a view of scientific investigation converging on the truth (Kuhn 1970). Social constructivists maintain that scientific "facts" are social products arising from the interests and social networks of the participating scientists (Woolgar 1988). Whatever plausibility antirealism might have for exotic theories such as quantum mechanics, the roles of instruments and experiments in the ulcers and bacteria case support medical realism. I argue that ulcers and *H. pylori* bacteria are real entities independent of any mental and social constructions and that the theoretical claim that *H. pylori* is an important causal factor in ulcers can be accepted as true (see also chapter 14).

Empiricists can accept the reality of ulcers, since lesions are observable by the naked eye and stomach ulcers were identified in autopsies long before the microscope was invented. But bacteria cannot be observed without a microscope. Van Fraassen (1980) denies that scientists see through a microscope: His strict empiricism would prevent him from accepting as true the claim that bacteria exist. More plausibly, Hacking (1983 [chapter 11]) notes that very difficult physical processes, such as the diffraction of light for optical microscopes and the transmission of electrons for electron microscopes, yield identical results. Denying the reality of bacteria and other structures observed through microscopes, he argues, would make the common results of the different physical processes a "preposterous coincidence." The thousands of articles published on *H. pylori* reflect their authors' experiences of observing bacteria through optical and electron microscopes, experiences made even more shareable by published photographs such as Figure 5.1. The empiricist has no grounds for elevating unaided sense experience above the observational practice of microscopists: Like ordinary observation, microscopy is not error free, but it has a high degree of reliability shown by intersubjective agreement. *H. pylori* can be seen, even if it takes a microscope to do so.

Conceptualism is sometimes a useful antidote to a too simple empiricism, when it recognizes that understanding the world goes well beyond sense experience. But it can err in the other direction by downgrading the role of experimentation in scientific change. The relation of hypothesis and experiment is reciprocal, involving a kind of feedback loop in which experimental results suggest hypotheses, hypotheses suggest experiments, and so on. Experimental data are not theory independent, but they are not completely theory dependent either. Endoscopy and microscopy revealed gastric spiral bacteria even to researchers who thought that Warren and Marshall were wrong. The conceptual structures described in chapter 3 do not determine what researchers will detect with their instruments. Some of Marshall's experiments—for example, the early attempt to develop an animal model of disease production by *H. pylori*—were not successful. Even more remarkable, some researchers who set out to refute his claims about the link between bacteria and ulcers produced experiments that confirmed those claims. Scientists' investigations of nature depend heavily on the conceptual structures with which they design experiments, but experiments often display a recalcitrance to expectations that cannot be explained if one thinks of nature only as a mental construction.

Similarly, it is implausible to view the bacterial theory of ulcers wholly as a social construction. Chapter 6 describes various social processes such as collaboration, communication, and consensus that were important to the development and acceptance of the new ideas of this theory. But these social processes operated in concert not only with the psychological processes in the minds of researchers but also with the physical processes by which scientists used instruments to interact with the world. Financial, ideological, medical, or other interests do not suffice to enable medical researchers to see what they want to see through a microscope or to obtain the biopsy samples they want to obtain with an endoscope. Using commonly accepted instrumental techniques and experimental methods, scientists achieved consensus in part because of physical interaction with a world not generated by their mental and social processes. Anyone who believes that *H. pylori* and the diseases it causes are pure social or mental constructions might receive a useful dose of reality by replicating Marshall's self-experiment.

Note that the emphasis on instruments and experiments in this chapter is not an explanation for scientific change that competes with the cognitive explanations given in chapters 3 and 4. The use of instruments in observation and the design and conduct of experiments all depend on mental representations for diseases and microbes. Interacting with the world depends on thinking, just as thinking depends on interacting with the world.

In sum, the ulcers and bacteria case has several aspects that support a realist interpretation: reliability of instruments, experimental recalcitrance, and causal efficacy. Unless one accepts as true the claims that *H. pylori* bacteria inhabit the stomach and can cause ulcers, there is no plausible explanation of why so many scientists have been able to observe the bacteria with microscopes, of why experimenters sometimes do not obtain the results they want, and of why antibiotics are such an effective cure for many cases of ulcers. I return to the defense of medical realism at the end of chapter 14.

Like most scientists, medical researchers do *not* spend most of their time theorizing. They devote immense efforts to designing, conducting, and analyzing the results of experiments. Scientific experiments often involve instruments of varying degrees of complexity, from the multibillion dollar accelerators needed for research in high-energy physics to the multimillion dollar brain scanning devices increasingly used in neuroscience to the computers used by cognitive psychologists to measure reaction times. In all these fields, there is great epistemological significance in the recalcitrance of nature, which often fails to provide researchers with the experimental results they expect. This recalcitrance, and the role of instruments and experimental design in enabling researchers to manipulate natural occurrences, renders implausible any attempt to construe the world purely as a mental or social construction. Understanding scientific change requires paying attention not only to the minds and social interactions of scientists but also to the physical activities by which these scientists intervene in the world and extract information from it. The development and acceptance of the bacterial theory of ulcers depended crucially on the use of instruments such as microscopes and endoscopes that are needed to observe bacteria and ulcers, and also on a series of experiments that were required to demonstrate a causal relation between *H. pylori* infection and gastric ulcers. Scientific change is equally a mental, physical, and social process.

SUMMARY

The discovery and evaluation of the bacterial theory of ulcers depended on several kinds of scientific instruments, particularly microscopes and endoscopes. Several kinds of experiments contributed to the development and acceptance of the theory, particularly intervention studies that showed that eradicating *H. pylori* usually cures peptic ulcers. Experimentation and theory interacted to produce good evidence in support of the claim that bacteria cause ulcers. This case therefore supports medical realism, the view that diseases and their causes are real and not just mental or social constructions. The physical processes of instrument use and experimentation are complementary to the mental processes of discovery and acceptance.

CHAPTER 6

Ulcers and Bacteria: Social Interactions

THIS CHAPTER describes several social processes that in part explain how the theory that most peptic ulcers are caused by *Helicobacter pylori* came to be formed and eventually accepted. First, research in this area, as with most current science, is highly collaborative, involving multiple scientists working together. Second, spread of the new ideas about ulcers required the communication of these ideas through the medical community by various means, including personal contact, conferences, and publications. Third, the growing consensus that ulcers are caused by bacteria is the result of various social processes, including a Consensus Development Panel meeting convened by the U.S. National Institutes of Health (NIH) in 1994. I describe more briefly other social aspects of scientific change, including the funding of medical research and the role of pharmaceutical companies.

COLLABORATION

A glance at science journals such as *Nature, Science*, and *Physical Review Letters* shows that the vast majority of scientific papers today are coauthored and reflect a variety of kinds of collaboration among scientists. Similarly, most medical research today is collaborative. For example, of the forty-four research articles in the July to September 1995 issues of *Lancet*, only one is single-authored, and the average number of authors per article is greater than seven. Similarly, research on the bacterial theory of ulcers has been highly collaborative, as I detail by describing the joint work of Robin Warren, Barry Marshall, and other researchers.

Warren and Marshall

One obvious reason why scientists collaborate is that there are research projects that require more expertise than any one individual possesses. Warren, a pathologist at Royal Perth Hospital, discovered gastric spiral bacteria in stomach biopsies in 1979. He was unable to investigate their clinical significance on his own, however, since that investigation required expertise in gastroenterology. In 1981, Marshall was a trainee in internal medicine, and the chief of gastroenterology, Tom Waters, suggested that Marshall carry out clinical research on the medical significance of Warren's bacteria. This research required both gastroenterology, to identify cases of gastric disease and take biopsies, and pathology, to determine the presence or absence of bacteria in the biopsies.

The first publication on ulcers and bacteria by Warren and Marshall has a curious structure. Under a common title, "Unidentified curved bacilli on gastric epithelium in active chronic gastritis," *Lancet* published two separate letters, one by Warren and one by Marshall (Warren and Marshall 1983). Warren's letter described work on the bacteria that he had conducted before beginning collaboration with Marshall. Marshall and Warren subsequently published several joint papers that reflected their continuing collaboration. The two letters are usually cited as one publication. Goodwin and Worsley (1993, p. 3) state that the unusual format was suggested by the electron microscopist J. A. Armstrong because Warren and Marshall could not agree on the wording of a joint letter. However, according to Warren (personal communication 1996), the letters were kept separate because the first one reflected work he had done alone; the second letter, which lists Marshall as author, described their joint work.

Early Experiments

The 1982 study, which first revealed an association between bacterial infection and peptic ulcers, was a collaborative effort that required both gastroenterology and pathology (Marshall and Warren 1984). At the end of this paper, Marshall and Warren (1984, p. 1314) thank a host of people who provided various kinds of assistance:

> We thank Dr. T. E. Waters, Dr. C. R. Sanderson, and the gastroenterology unit staff for the biopsies, Miss Helen Royce and Dr. D. I. Annear for the microbiology studies, Mr. Peter Rogers and Dr. L. Sly for supplying the G & C data, Dr. J. A. Armstrong for the electron microscopy, Dr. R. Glancy for reviewing slides, Miss Joan Bot for the silver stains, Mrs. Rose Rendell of Raine Medical Statistics Unit UWA, and Ms. Maureen Humphries, secretary, and, for travel support, Fremantle Hospital.

Notice the wealth of expertise required for the study: gastroenterology, microbiology, microscopy, and statistics. All these specialties require years of intense training, so no individual researcher could have conducted the 1982 study alone.

Similarly, the 1984 attempt to fulfil Koch's postulates for bacteria and gastritis by Marshall's self-experiment required a team of researchers (Marshall et al. 1985). This paper lists the specialties of the authors as follows:

Barry J. Marshall, registrar in microbiology
David B. McGechie, microbiologist
Ross J. Clancy, pathologist
John A. Armstrong, electron microscopist

Marshall's self-administration of bacteria would have been uninformative without the assistance of various specialists to help determine whether the bacteria had infected his stomach. That additional help was useful for this project is clear from the acknowledgments (Marshall et al. 1985, p. 439):

We wish to thank Dr. J. R. Warren for advice on the historical aspects; Dr. I. G. Hislop for performing the gastroscopies; Mr. N. Nokes for the cultures; and S. H. Wee (EM) and J. E. Holdsworth for the histological preparations.

Whereas the 1982 experiment was performed in one hospital, Royal Perth, the 1984 experiment required collaboration across two organizations. When it was conducted, Marshall, McGechie, and Clancy all were in the department of microbiology at Fremantle Hospital, whereas Armstrong was at Royal Perth. Note also how the need for collaborators often corresponds to the need for expertise with different instruments. This project required gastroenterologists for expertise with gastroscopy, pathologists for expertise with microscopes, microbiologists for expertise with stains and cultures, and an expert whose profession was defined by his instrument, the electron microscope.

Treatment Experiments

The need for collaboration intensified with the studies begun in 1985 to determine whether eradication of bacteria is an effective treatment for duodenal ulcers. The Marshall et al. study (1988) has no fewer than nine coauthors drawn from four medical specialties: gastroenterology (Barry Marshall, Raymond Murray, Thomas E. Waters, Christopher R. Sanderson), microbiology (C. Stewart Goodwin, Elizabeth D. Blincow), histopathology (J. Robin Warren), and pharmacy (Stephen J. Blackbourn). The ninth researcher, Michael Phillips, is listed as being at Curtin University in Perth. The acknowledgments thank several other personnel for help with endoscopies. The seven year follow-up to determine the long-term benefits of *H. pylori* eradication required a similarly broad range of expertise, although the researchers were different except for Warren and Marshall (Forbes et al. 1994). Clearly, experimental demonstration that antibiotics can cure ulcers required cooperation across medical specialties.

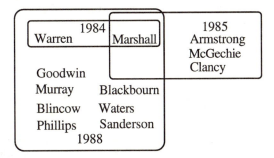

Figure 6.1. Research teams, as shown by the authorship of Marshall and Warren (1984), Marshall et al. (1985), and Marshall et al. (1988).

In chapter 4, I cited five additional papers that provide convincing evidence that the use of antibiotics to eradicate *H. pylori* cures gastric or duodenal ulcers. All five papers are coauthored, with an average of more than five authors per paper. For example, the researchers who collaborated with David Graham (e.g., Graham et al. 1992) include epidemiologists, pediatricians, and pathologists as well as gastroenterologists. One paper that found an association between *H. pylori* infection and gastric cancer lists as its author the "EUROGAST Study Group," which has more than two dozen members spread across many countries and institutions (EUROGAST Study Group 1993).

It is therefore obvious that the research that produced the evidential support for the bacterial theory of ulcers is not the product of individual minds working in isolation but of the cooperative work of many teams of scientists. Figure 6.1 shows some of the social connections that contributed to the work of Marshall and Warren, grouped according to coauthorship. Such interconnections are typical of research in the natural sciences as well as in some social sciences, such as psychology. Hence, the interactions of researchers in producing and interpreting experimental research must be taken into consideration in any adequate account of scientific change. In the terminology of social network analysis, collaboration can be understood as a kind of affiliation network, and Figure 6.1 can be interpreted as a hypergraph (Wasserman and Faust 1994). A much more complicated graph would be needed to display all the relevant collaborations.

Philosophy of science is concerned not only with how science is done but also with how it should be done. My conclusions concerning the importance of collaboration to the ulcers and bacteria case are both descriptive and normative. Descriptively, we must notice that collaboration did occur; normatively, it is clear that scientific research concerning peptic ulcers and *H. pylori* would have been much less effective, efficient, and illuminating without collaborations among pathologists, gastroenterologists, microbiologists, and other personnel. As with much other research in contemporary science, collaboration not only facilitates scientific change but is essential to it. See chapter 11 for further normative analysis of collaboration.

COMMUNICATION

Scientific change requires not only the production of research but also its communication to other researchers. This section outlines the role of four kinds of communication—personal contacts, conferences, journals, and the public press—in the development and dissemination of the bacterial theory of ulcers.

Personal Contacts

The spread of new ideas often depends on personal interactions. In 1981, Marshall heard about Warren's observations of gastric spiral bacteria, because Waters suggested that Marshall help Warren investigate the bacteria. Personal contacts were also important in arranging the first international presentation of the results of the 1982 study that first found an association between ulcers and bacteria. McGechie, a microbiologist at Fremantle Hospital, had received an invitation to the International Workshop on *Campylobacter* Infections, and he suggested to Marshall that he submit his findings to that meeting (Marshall 1989). McGechie provided Marshall with the home telephone number of Martin Skirrow in Worcester, England. After a phone conversation, Marshall mailed Skirrow some isolates of the newly cultured bacteria.

Once the new ideas about bacteria and ulcers began to gain acceptance, the main researchers, such as Marshall and Graham were in great demand for speaking engagements, another kind of personal contact. In 1996, Marshall was booked eighteen months in advance for personal appearances.

Conferences

The first public presentation of the results of the 1982 study was the local meeting of the Royal Australian College of Physicians in 1982 (Marshall 1989). Marshall's submission to the 1983 meeting of the Australian Gastroenterological Society was rejected, but in contrast, his presentation at the International Workshop on *Campylobacter* Infections in Brussels in 1983 prompted substantial interest in researchers from several countries. Subsequent conferences and their published proceedings (e.g., Blaser 1989) provided important avenues of communication.

The hypothesis that the gastric spiral bacteria caused ulcers had a much more positive initial reception from medical microbiologists than from gastro-enterologists, who had preexisting ideas about acidity as the major causal factor in ulcers. Marshall and Warren's (1984) report of their 1982 study was not immediately accepted by the editors of *Lancet*, who had received negative evaluations from experts invited to review the report. But as a result of the 1983 meeting in Brussels, a number of microbiologists such as Martin Blaser began finding the bacteria in patients with gastritis and ulcers. The growing recognition of the importance of Marshall and Warren's research made gastro-enterologists take the finding more seriously. Using a football analogy, we might describe the acceptance of the bacterial theory ulcers as a kind of "epistemic end run": a direct assault on gastroenterology was unsuccessful because of entrenched ideas in that field, but an indirect pursuit of the new ideas was possible via microbiology.

It must be recognized, however, that in the mid-1980s the evidence for the claim that *H. pylori* causes peptic ulcers was meager. Even gastroenterologists who were interested in the new hypothesis viewed it as lacking in scientific support. They were annoyed by conference presentations that aggressively pushed the hypothesis in the absence of careful experiments that supported the causal claim. By the 1990s, however, such experiments had been conducted by various researchers, and conference discussion shifted from the question of whether *H. pylori* causes ulcers to how it does so and how it can be eradicated.

Journals

Warren and Marshall published their 1983 and 1984 communications, as well as the 1988 article on treatment of duodenal ulcers, in *Lancet*, the most widely read British medical journal. The subsequent dramatic growth of interest in ulcers and bacteria is clear in Figure 6.2, which shows that by 1989 there were well over one hundred papers published on the topic. Most of the papers published in the 1990s that provided substantial evidence that eradication of *H. pylori* cures peptic ulcers were published in *Lancet*, although some also appeared in the *New England Journal of Medicine* and *Annals of Internal Medicine* (see chapter 4 for references). Thousands of articles about *H. pylori* and its role of disease have been published, and a new *Journal of Helicobacter* is forthcoming, edited by David Graham.

Unlike most scientific journals, medical journals such as *Lancet* and the *New England Journal of Medicine* publish editorials along with research reports. The editorials allow experts in a field to comment on the clinical significance of recent findings. David Graham, for example, wrote an editorial for the *New England Journal of Medicine* (1993) that discussed recent studies and

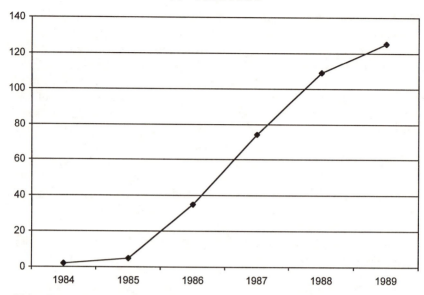

Figure 6.2. Growth in the number of journal articles on the role of *Helicobacter pylori* in peptic ulcer disease and gastritis. Adapted from *Science Watch, 1, 7*, published by the Institute for Scientific Information.

argued that *H. pylori* infection is the most common cause of peptic ulcer and accounts for the majority of cases. Because such editorials are concise and less technical than research reports, they may have a substantial impact on belief change in medical researchers and physicians not directly involved with the topic.

Popular Media

Although in recent years the bacterial theory of ulcers has received enormous support in the medical journals, some physicians are still treating ulcer patients with traditional antacids. The communication of research results to physicians is often delayed, since many of them do not routinely read reports of clinical trials but instead obtain their information indirectly through newsletters and drug company announcements (see Figure 12.3). On the other hand, some patients have heard about the new results more quickly thanks to reports on Marshall's work that have appeared in the popular press, in publications such as the *New York Times*, the *Washington Post, Consumer Reports*, and the *New Yorker*. Television shows describing the breakthroughs have been broadcast in Australia, England, and Canada. Because peptic ulcers affect such a large proportion (10%) of the population, it is not surprising that reports of a new cure have received popular attention. More surprising is the fact that in some instances patients have had to bring the new treatments to the attention of their physicians, rather than vice versa. In 1996, the American Gastroenterological Association conducted a major media campaign to bring awareness of the new treatments for ulcers to the public at large.

CONSENSUS

In most scientific fields, consensus evolves intangibly, as myriad scientists come to accept new hypotheses. Consensus may slowly become evident in the converging statements of review articles and textbooks, but there is no central social mechanism that produces a consensus. In medical research, the need for a consensus is much more acute, since hypotheses such as the bacterial theory of ulcers have direct consequences for the treatment of patients. In February 1994, the NIH convened a conference in Washington, D.C., to examine the claim that peptic ulcers are caused by *H. pylori*.

Since 1977, the NIH has conducted a Consensus Development Conference Program whose purpose is produce consensus statements on important and controversial statements in medicine. The NIH's Web site describes the program as follows:

> NIH Consensus Development Conferences are convened to evaluate available scientific information and resolve safety and efficacy issues related to biomedical technology. The resultant NIH Consensus Statements are intended to advance understanding of the technology or issue in question and to be useful to health professionals and the public. NIH Consensus Statements are prepared by a non advocate, non-Federal panel of experts, based on (1) presentations by investigators working in areas relevant to the consensus questions during a 2-day public session; (2) questions and statements from conference attendees during open discussion periods that are part of the public session; and (3) closed deliberations by the panel during the remainder of the second day and morning of the third. This statement is an independent report of the panel and is not a policy statement of the NIH or the Federal Government. (available at http://text.nlm.nih.gov/nih/upload-v3/About/about.html)

The 1994 consensus development conference on *H. pylori* in peptic ulcer disease was the ninety-fourth sponsored by the NIH.

In accord with NIH guidelines, this conference was organized around several groups of people. First, a planning committee was established, chaired by Tadataka Yamada, Chair of the Department of Internal Medicine at the University of Michigan. The planning committee chair is required to be a knowledgeable and highly regarded medical figure who is not identified with strong advocacy of the conference topic or with relevant research. The fifteen other members of the planning committee included researchers who were by then advocates of the bacterial theory of ulcers, including Blaser, Graham, and Marshall, but it also included experts on digestive diseases who were not so directly involved. The consensus development panel consisted of fourteen people who were chosen for various kinds of expertise and who were specifically not identified with advocacy or promotional positions regarding the issues to be resolved by the conference.

Presentations to the panel were made by twenty-two researchers who were advocates for and against the claim that *H. pylori* bacteria are a causal factor in peptic ulcers. Blaser, Graham, and Marshall were among those who argued in support of that claim, but more skeptical presentations had such titles as "Limitations of the *Helicobacter pylori* hypothesis" and "Current uncertainties about the impact of *Helicobacter pylori* on the complications of peptic ulcer disease." By 1994, however, the case for bacterial involvement in ulcers was strong, and most of the speakers at the consensus conference supported it. On February 9, 1994, the panel presented its statement concluding that ulcer patients with *H. pylori* infection require treatment with antimicrobial agents. This statement was later published in the widely read *Journal of the American Medical Association* (National Institutes of Health Consensus Development Panel 1994).

The NIH panel was a formal version of a process that often occurs informally in science, when relatively disinterested researchers can constitute a kind of jury for settling scientific controversies. Kim (1994), for example, describes how early in this century medical personnel provided a kind of neutral jury to evaluate disputes concerning the plausibility of Mendelian genetics, which had both advocates and critics. Similarly, the hypothesis proposed in 1980 that dinosaur extinction was caused by an asteroid striking the earth had vehement advocates and critics; but there were also many informed members of the scientific community who were not directly involved in the controversy and who were sufficiently well informed to provide objective assessment of the evidence. Science benefits both from a diversity of approaches, when some researchers pursue new ideas even when there is limited empirical support for them, and from the social process by which researchers with no stake in or bias against those ideas provide an informed evaluation of them.

The 1994 NIH conference was only one of the social mechanisms that encouraged increased acceptance of the bacterial theory of ulcers. Some researchers and physicians learned about the emerging evidence for the theory from conferences, journals, and personal contacts. Consensus was not universal: John Graham (1995) rejected the claim that *H. pylori* has been shown to be the primary cause of peptic ulcers. As of 1996, although some physicians were still treating patients with antacids instead of antibiotics, gastroenterologists were involved in organized efforts to disseminate treatment information to a broad audience of physicians and patients. Chapter 12 discusses the 1997 consensus panel meetings that took place in the United States, Canada, and elsewhere.

ORGANIZATIONS AND FUNDING

The social processes that in part produce scientific change involve organizations as well as individuals. In medical research, the U.S. NIH plays a direct role in encouraging consensus about treatments. Other organizations, however, were important in the earlier development of the bacterial theory of ulcers, which depended on hospitals, universities, drug companies, and other funding agencies.

Warren and Marshall's initial collaboration took place at the Royal Perth Hospital. Their early research does not cite any special funding sources but was supported by the resources of the Royal Perth and Fremantle Hospitals (Marshall et al. 1985; Marshall and Warren 1984; Warren and Marshall 1983). Subsequent larger scale trials required greater resources, and the 1985 to 1987 research on eradication of *H. pylori* used funds from the National Health and Medical Research Council of Australia, the Royal Perth Hospital General Fund, Gist Brocades, and Pfizer (Marshall et al. 1988). After Marshall left Australia in 1986, he conducted his research at the University of Virginia Health Sciences Center. In 1996, his Web page included a disclaimer that indicated he was consulting with and accepting honoraria from Astra-Merck, Abbott, Glaxo-Wellcome, Eli-Lilley, Pfizer, Procter and Gamble, and many other medical companies (available at http://vianet.net.au/bjmrshll/index.html; see also http://www.helico.com/). In addition, Marshall reported holding stock in several pharmaceutical and diagnostic companies and having an interest in Tri-Med Specialties Inc. and Meretek, which are companies developing urea breath tests for *H. pylori*.

Clinical trials are expensive and usually require funding by pharmaceutical companies that have an interest in showing that a new drug is effective. Bradley (1993, p. 153) reports a survey that found that eighty-nine percent of trials that were supported by the pharmaceutical industry had positive results in favor of a new treatment but that only sixty-one percent of trials not so supported found positive results. Because *H. pylori* infections can be cured with combinations of generic antibiotics in which no drug company has a proprietary interest, funding for research on this topic has been primarily obtained from other sources. Many of the early experiments on ulcers and *H. pylori* were conducted by interested researchers using funds redirected from other projects. The makers of Zantac and Tagamet, two of the most lucrative drugs ever produced, have an interest against the new treatment of ulcers, which can actually eradicate the disease, but the drug companies mounted no resistance to the new theory of ulcers. Zantac and Tagamet have recently become available in the United States without a prescription, allowing people with gastric distress to alleviate their symptoms without consulting physicians about the possible presence of *H. pylori* infections. In the United States, pharmaceutical companies have recently received approval for drugs that combine antacid and antibiotic treatments. These should make it easier for physicians to know what to prescribe to their ulcer patients.

In the United States and Canada, conservative government funding agencies were slow to appreciate the medical importance of *H. pylori.* The role of *H. pylori* in ulcers, gastric cancer, and other diseases is a socioeconomic as well as a medical issue, since government health providers stand to save substantial amounts of money by eradicating *H. pylori* rather than pursuing traditional antacid treatment (O'Brien et al. 1996).

SCIENCE AS A SOCIAL PROCESS

My account of the social processes affecting the new theory of ulcers is incompatible both with traditional philosophy of science, which tends to ignore the social altogether, and with some aspects of modern sociology of science, which tends to give the social an exclusive role in explaining scientific change. Philosophy of science claims to reach normative conclusions about how science should be done, but philosophical research informed by history and psychology shows how descriptive studies can inform normative conclusions (Thagard 1988 [chapter 7]). Similarly, descriptive studies of the social contributors to scientific development can feed into normative conclusions. It is obvious, for example, that collaboration was a positive contributor to the emergence of the bacterial theory of ulcers, since the critical experimental studies could not have been performed without combining the expertise of gastroenterologists, pathologists, microbiologists, and others. Normatively, therefore, we can conclude that collaboration is a social process that contributes to the development of scientific knowledge. Another contributor is the organization of the NIH Consensus Development Conferences, in which a panel of experts with no special interests in the issue convenes to hear diverse presentations and reach an impartial recommendation about treatment. As sociologists have pointed out, scientists approach their research with diverse interests and social contexts that undoubtedly affect their work, but institutions such as the NIH panel provide a relatively impartial forum for evaluating competing claims. The panel is a more concentrated and organized form of what takes place in journals through the procedure of peer review.

While noticing the importance of social processes such as collaboration, communication, consensus, and funding to scientific research, it is important not to succumb to the slogan that science is a social construction. Proponents of that slogan tend to ignore the psychological processes of theory construction and acceptance (see chapters 3 and 4) as well as the physical processes of interaction with the world via instruments and experiments (see chapter 5). Undoubtedly, interests and social networks abound in the ulcers case as in other episodes in the history of science. But explaining scientific change solely on the basis of social factors is as patently inadequate as are purely logical and psychological explanations.

Latour (1988, p. 229) says that science is politics by other means. He depicts research as a Machiavellian series of trials of strength in which scientists attempt to recruit allies to vanquish their foes. A Latourian history of the bacterial theory of ulcers would ignore the cognitive processes of scientists, since Latour (1988, p. 218) says that we do not think, only write. It would also misconstrue the role of instruments and experiments, as when Latour (1988, p. 73) explains Pasteur's laboratory work by saying: "To win, we have only to bring the enemy to where we are sure we will be the stronger. A researcher like Pasteur was strongest in the laboratory." This is nonsense; microbiologists go to the laboratory because it enables them to study organisms under controlled conditions with the appropriate instruments. Of course, science does have a political side, evident in the operations of funding agencies, consensus panels, and other social operations, such as Marshall's working with microbiologists in the face of opposition from many gastroenterologists. But science also has cognitive and experimental sides that must figure in explanations of scientific change.

Chapter 1 presented a Social Explanation Schema for belief acquisition that attributed scientists' belief changes to social interests and power relations. I could have gone into more detail about the various interests involved in this case, such as the interests of gastroenterologists to maintain lucrative practices and the interests of drug companies to protect markets for profitable drugs. Undoubtedly, Marshall and the early advocates of the bacterial theory of ulcers had to struggle against the power of the medical establishment. But it is striking that a decade of experimental research sufficed to subordinate these factors to the cognitive and practical interests of gastroenterologists who have used scientific evidence to determine the best course of treatment for their patients.

CONCLUSION

What causes scientific change? This question is clearly at least as complex as the question of what causes ulcers. In the latter case, although the eradication studies show that *H. pylori* infection is probably the most important cause of peptic ulcers, a full account of the etiology of ulcers has to take into account a wealth of other factors that help to explain why only some of the people who have bacterial infections develop ulcers. Future research on the operation of the digestive and immune systems should start to fill in some of the answers. The causal mechanisms by which *H. pylori* produces ulcers are already becoming better understood (e.g., Olbe et al. 1996). Similarly, a complex of psychological, physical, and social mechanisms were responsible for the development and acceptance of the bacterial theory of ulcers. One of the most important mechanisms, I contend, is the psychological process of assessment of explanatory coherence (see chapter 4). Scientific change is in part the changes in scientists' minds, and explanatory coherence provides the most psychologically and historically plausible account of belief revision now available. But a more complete view of the causes of scientific change is presented in chapter 14, after a more general discussion of the social processes involved in the growth of medical knowledge (chapters 11 to 13).

Although it has been convenient to discuss the bacterial theory of ulcers in terms of mind, nature, and society, we must not forget the interactions among these elements. Mind affects nature through the mental processes crucial to the use of instruments and the design of experiments, while nature affects mind by producing observations and experimental results that may or may not conform with expectations. Society affects mind through the goals and interests that motivate scientists and through the organizations and social networks that make modern science possible, while mind affects society when organizations are affected by the discoveries of individuals. Society affects nature through the contributions of needs, organizations, and networks to experimental research, while nature affects society when scientific organizations contribute to new discoveries that arise from interactions with the world.

One aspect of mind that I have neglected in these chapters is personality. Personal characteristics such as aggressiveness, tenacity, and conservatism were undoubtedly of some importance in the roles that different researchers played in the ulcers and bacteria case. This case does not support the claim that scientific change is primarily produced by later born children (Sulloway 1996), since Warren and Marshall are both eldest children. Gender and nationality also do not seem to have been factors in the ulcers case.

My account of the emergence since the mid-1980s of major views about the causes of ulcers has described science as a complex system. The system is simultaneously psychological (involving individual scientists' cognitive processes for discovery and acceptance), physical (requiring scientists to interact with the natural world using instruments and experiments), and social (involving the interaction of scientists with each other). The result is a rich instantiation of the Cognitive-Social Explanation Schema presented in chapter 1. Only by attending to all these aspects of the growth of knowledge can we fully explain scientific change. Contrary to the traditional and postmodern views, science is neither just a matter of logic nor just a matter of politics. Logic contributes to the development of science when theories are evaluated on the basis of their explanatory coherence, and science is political when researchers agitate for acceptance and funding of their favorite ideas. But logic and politics both operate within a much larger system of psychological, physical, and social processes. Chapter 14 provides further discussion of the complexities of science.

SUMMARY

The discovery and evaluation of the bacterial theory of ulcers depended on social as well as psychological and physical processes. Collaboration among researchers with complementary areas of expertise was essential for experimental and theoretical progress. Communication of ideas among researchers involved personal contacts, conferences, and journals. The 1994 meeting of the NIH Consensus Development Panel was an important forum for evaluating the status of the bacterial theory of ulcers, and the panel's published decision had a substantial impact on general opinion in the field. Organizations such as hospitals, universities, and pharmaceutical companies were important for the funding of research. Despite the importance of social processes in this case, it would be an exaggeration to describe the bacterial theory of ulcers as socially constructed, since its development and acceptance were the result of a complex system that was psychological and physical as well as social.

Part Three

COGNITIVE PROCESSES

CHAPTER 7

Causes, Correlations, and Mechanisms

I NOW examine in more detail some of the cognitive processes involved in the development of the bacterial theory of ulcers and in other cases of the growth of medical knowledge. This chapter concerns how causes are inferred from correlations and other information about mechanisms and alternative causes. It first discusses the inference from correlation to causation, integrating recent psychological discussions of causal reasoning with epidemiological approaches to understanding disease causation. In addition to the bacterial theory of ulcers, this chapter considers the evolution over the past several decades of ideas about the causes of cancer, particularly lung cancer. Both of these developments involved progression from observed correlations to accepted causal hypotheses (e.g., bacteria cause ulcers, smoking causes cancer), followed by an increased understanding of the mechanisms by which the causes produce the diseases. There is much more to causal reasoning than simply noticing that two factors are associated with each other. I describe how causal mechanisms represented by causal networks can contribute to reasoning that involves correlation and causation. An understanding of causation and causal mechanisms provides the basis for presentation of a model of medical explanation as causal network instantiation.

CORRELATION AND CAUSES

Explanation of why people get a particular disease usually begins by noticing associations between the disease and possible causal factors. For example, the bacterial theory of ulcers originated when Barry Marshall and Robin Warren noticed an association between duodenal ulcer and infection with *Helicobacter pylori* (see chapter 3). They were aware that their study did not establish a cause-and-effect relation between bacteria and ulcers, but they took it as evidence that the bacteria were etiologically related to the ulcers and undertook studies to determine whether eradicating the ulcers would cure the bacteria (see chapters 4 and 5).

A similar progression from correlation to causation has taken place with various kinds of cancer. Over two thousand years ago, Hippocrates described cancers of the skin, stomach, breast, and other body locations and held that cancer is caused, like all diseases, by an imbalance of bodily humors, particularly an excess of black bile. In the eighteenth century, rough correlations were noticed between cancers and various practices: using snuff and nose cancer, pipe smoking and lip cancer, chimney sweeping and scrotum cancer, and being a nun and breast cancer (Proctor 1995, pp. 27–28). The perils of causal reasoning are shown by the inferences of the Italian physician Bernardino Ramazzini, who concluded in 1713 that the increased incidence of breast cancer in nuns was caused by their sexual abstinence, rather than by their not having children. Early in the twentieth century, it was shown that cancers can be induced in laboratory animals by radiation and coal tar.

Lung cancer rates increased significantly in Great Britain and the United States during the first half of the twentieth century, correlating with increase in smoking. Carefully controlled studies, however, began to appear only in the 1950s (Hennekens and Buring 1987, p. 44). In one classic study conducted in England, 649 male and sixty female patients with lung cancer were matched to an equal number of control patients of the same age and sex. For both men and women, there was a strong correlation between lung cancer and smoking, particularly heavy smoking. By 1964, when the U.S. Surgeon General's Report asserted a causal link between lung cancer and smoking, there had been twenty-nine controlled studies performed in numerous countries that showed a high statistical association between lung cancer and smoking. Although the exact mechanism by which smoking causes cancer was not known, more than two hundred different compounds had been identified in cigarette smoke that were known carcinogens.

To grasp how disease explanations work, we need to understand what correlations are, what causes are, and how correlations can provide evidence for causes. Patricia Cheng's (1997) Power PC theory of how people infer causal powers from probabilistic information provides a useful starting point. She proposes that when scientists and other people infer the causes of events, they use an intuitive notion of causal power to explain observed correlations. She characterizes correlation (covariation) in terms of probabilistic contrasts: how much more probable an effect is with a cause than without a cause. The association between an effect e and a possible cause c can be measured by the following equation:

$$\Delta P_c = P(e/c) - P(e/\sim c)$$

The probability of e given c (e/c) is calculated minus the probability of e without c ($e/\sim c$). However, in contrast to many philosophers who try to give a purely probabilistic account of causality, she introduces an additional notion of the *power* of a cause c to produce an effect e, p_c, which is the probability with which c produces e when c is present. Whereas $P(e/c)$ is an observable frequency, p_c is a theoretical entity that is hypothesized to explain frequencies, just as theoretical entities such as electrons and molecules are hypothesized to explain observations in physics. In Cheng's account, causes are used to provide theoretical explanations of correlations, just as theories such as the kinetic theory of gases are used to explain laws such as those linking observed properties of gases (i.e., pressure, volume, temperature).

Terminologically, I take *correlation* to be interchangeable with *covariation* and *statistical association*. Correlations are not always measured by the statistical formula for coefficient of correlation, which applies only to linear relationships. As with Cheng's theory, the work of Peng and Reggia (1990, p. 101f) involves "probabilistic causal models" that rely not on conditional probabilities of the form P(effect/disease) but on "conditional causal probabilities" of the form P(disease causes effect/disease). Both probabilistic and causal power ideas have a long history in philosophy. On probabilistic causality, see, for example, Eells (1991), Shafer (1996), and Suppes (1970). On causal powers, see, for example, Cartwright (1989) and Harré and Madden (1975).

According to Cheng (1997), a causal power p_c is a probability, but what kind of probability? Philosophers have debated whether probabilities are frequencies, logical relations, or subjective states, but the interpretation of probability that seems to fit best with Cheng's view is that a probability is a propensity, that is, a dispositional property of part of the world to produce a frequency of events in the long run. The causal power p_c cannot be immediately inferred from the observed frequency $P(e/c)$ or the contrast ΔP_c, because the effect e may be due to alternative causes. Celibate nuns get breast cancer more than non-nuns, but it is nonpregnancy rather than celibacy that is causally related to breast cancer. To estimate the causal power of c to produce e, we need to take into account alternative possible causes of e, designated collectively as a. If there are no alternative causes of e besides c, then $P(e/c) = p_c$, but they will normally not be equal if a is present and produces e in the presence of c, that is, if $P(a/c)*p_a > 0$, where p_a is the causal power of a to produce c and * indicates multiplication. In the simple case which a occurs independently of c, Cheng shows that p_c can be estimated using the following equation:

$$p_c = \Delta P_c \,/\, 1 - P(a)*p_a$$

The causal relation between e and c can thus be assessed by considering positively the correlation between e and c and negatively the operation of other causes a. When these alternative causes do not occur independently of c, then ΔP_c may not reflect the causal status of c.

Cheng's characterization of the relation between correlations and causal powers fits well with epidemiologists' discussions of the problem of determining the causes of diseases. Her account also fits with the view of Chinn and Brewer (1996) that data interpretation is a matter of building mental models that include alternative explanations. According to Hennekens and Buring

TABLE 7.1

Framework for the Interpretation of an Epidemiological Study

A. Is there a valid statistical association?
  1. Is the association likely to be due to chance?
  2. Is the association likely to be due to bias?
  3. Is the association likely to be due to confounding?

B. Can this valid statistical association be judged as cause and effect?
  1. Is there a strong association?
  2. Is there biological credibility to the hypothesis?
  3. Is there consistency with other studies?
  4. Is the time sequence compatible?
  5. Is there evidence of a dose-response relationship?

Source: From Hennekens and Buring (1987, p. 45).

(1987, p. 30), a causal association is one in which a "change in the frequency or quality of an exposure or characteristic results in a corresponding change in the frequency of the disease or outcome of interest." Elwood (1988, p. 6) says that "a factor is a cause of an event if its operation increases the frequency of the event." These statements incorporate both ΔP_c, captured by the change in frequency, and the idea that the change in frequency is the result of the operation of the cause (i.e., a causal power). Further, epidemiologists stress that assessing whether the results of a study reveal a causal relation requires one to consider alternative explanations of the observed association, such as chance, bias in the design of the study, and confounding alternative causes (Table 4.1; see also Evans 1993; Susser 1973). Thus, the inference from correlation to cause must consider possible alternative causes, p_a.

Hennekens and Buring (1997) summarize their extensive discussion of epidemiological studies in the framework reproduced in Table 7.1. Questions A1 to A3 reflect the need to rule out alternative causes, and questions B1 and B3 reflect the desirability of high correlations, ΔP_c. Cheng's account of causal reasoning captures five of the eight questions relevant to assessing causal power, but the remaining three questions are beyond the scope of her model, which is restricted to induction from observable input. Hennekens and Buring (p. 40) state that "the belief in the existence of a cause and effect relationship is enhanced if there is a known or postulated biologic mechanism by which the exposure might reasonably alter the risk of the disease." Moreover (p. 42), "for a judgment of causality to be reasonable, it should be clear that the exposure of interest preceded the outcome by a period of time consistent with any proposed biologic mechanism." Thus, according to Hennekens and Buring, epidemiologists do and should ask mechanism-related questions about biological credibility and time sequence; this issue is discussed in the next section. Hennekens and Buring's last question concerns the existence of a dose-response relationship, that is, the observation of a gradient of risk associated with the degree of exposure. This relation is not just ΔP_c, the increased probability of having the disease given the cause, but rather the relation that being subjected to more of the cause produces more of the disease, as when heavy smokers get lung cancer more than light smokers.

Hennekens and Buring (1987) show how answers to the questions in Table 7.1 provide a strong case for a causal connection between smoking and lung cancer. Many studies have found a strong association between smoking and cancer, with a nine- to ten-fold increase in lung cancer among smokers (B1, B3), and the high statistical significance of the results makes it unlikely that the association is due to chance (A1). The conduct of the studies ruled out various sources of observation bias (A2), and researchers controlled for four potential confounding factors: age, sex, social class, and place of residence (A3). By 1959, cigarette smoke was known to contain more than two hundred different compounds that were known carcinogens, providing possible mechanisms to support the biological credibility of the hypothesis that smoking causes cancer (B2). Moreover, there was evidence of a temporal relationship between smoking and cancer, because people are more likely to get lung cancer if they have been smoking for a long time, whereas people who stop smoking dramatically drop their chances of getting cancer (B4). Finally, there is a significant dose-response relationship between smoking and lung cancer, in that the risk of developing lung cancer increases substantially with the number of cigarettes smoked per day and the duration of the habit.

The development of the bacterial theory of ulcers can be interpreted in terms of Cheng's theory of causality (1997) and Hennekens and Buring's framework for epidemiological investigation (1987). As described in chapter 4, when Marshall and Warren first proposed that peptic ulcers are caused by bacteria, most gastroenterologists were highly skeptical. They attributed the presence of bacteria in Warren's gastric biopsies to contamination, and they discounted the correlation between ulcers and bacterial infection as a likely result of chance or incorrect study design. Moreover, an alternative explanation that ulcers are caused by excess acidity was widely accepted because of the success of antacids in alleviating ulcer symptoms. But attitudes toward the ulcer hypothesis changed dramatically when numerous other researchers observed the bacteria in stomach samples, and especially when other research teams replicated Marshall and Warren's finding that eradicating *H. pylori* usually cures ulcers.

The key question is whether bacteria cause ulcers, which requires attributing to *H. pylori* the causal power to increase the occurrence of ulcers. Initial evidence for this attribution was the finding that people with the bacteria have ulcers more frequently than do those without the bacteria:

$$P(ulcers/bacteria) > P(ulcers/no\ bacteria)$$

The early studies, however, could not establish causality because they did not address the question of the existence of possible alternative causes for the ulcers. Whereas lung cancer investigators had to use case-control methods to rule out alternative causes by pairing up patients with lung cancers with similar patients without the disease, ulcer investigators could use the fact that *H. pylori* can be eradicated by antibiotics to perform a highly controlled experiment with one set of patients, comparing them before eradication and after. The eradication experiments described in chapters 3 and 4 show a high value for Δ*P*, *P(ulcers/bacteria)* – *P(ulcers/no bacteria)*, under circumstances in which no alternative causal factors such as stress, diet, and stomach acidity were varied.

Dose-response relationship has not been a factor in the conclusion that ulcers cause bacteria, since it is not easy to quantify how many bacteria inhabit a given patient's stomach. Time sequence is not much of an issue, since the common presence of the bacteria in children implies that people have the bacteria long before they develop ulcers. But biological credibility, concerning the mechanism by which bacterial infection might produce ulcers, has been the subject of much investigation, as I discuss in the next section. The correlation between ulcers and bacteria might be taken to suggest that ulcers cause bacterial infections, rather than the other way around. But the presence of bacteria is too widespread for this to be plausible: *P(bacteria/ulcers)* – *P(bacteria/ no ulcers)* is not high, since the bacteria are quite common, infecting as much as 50% of the population. Moreover, *H. pylori* bacteria were not found to be prominent on gastric ulcer borders, suggesting that the ulcers were not responsible for bacterial growth (see chapter 4).

In sum, much of the practice of physicians and epidemiologists in identifying the causes of diseases can be understood in terms of Cheng's theory, which states that causal powers are theoretical entities that are inferred on the basis of finding correlations and eliminating alternative causes. But mechanism considerations are also often relevant to assessing medical causality.

CAUSES AND MECHANISMS

What are mechanisms, and how does reasoning about them affect the inference of causes from correlations? A mechanism is a system of parts that operate or interact like those of a machine, transmitting forces, motion, and energy to one another. For millennia, humans have used simple machines such as levers, pulleys, inclined planes, screws, and wheels. More complicated machines can be built out of these simple ones, all of which transmit motion from one part to another by direct contact. In the sixteenth and seventeenth centuries, natural philosophers increasingly understood the world in terms of mechanisms, culminating with Newton's unified explanation of the motion of earthly and heav-

TABLE 7.2
Sketch of Some Important Mechanisms in Science

Science	Parts	Changes	Interactions
Physics	Objects such as sun and planets	Motion	Forces such as gravitation
Chemistry	Elements, molecules	Mass, energy	Reactions
Evolutionary biology	Organisms	New species	Natural selection
Genetics	Genes	Genetic transmission and alteration	Heredity, mutation, recombination,
Geology	Geological formations such as mountains	Creation and elimination of formations	Volcanoes, erosion
Plate tectonics	Continents	Motion such as continental drift	Floating, collision
Neuroscience	Neurons	Activation, synaptic connections	Electrochemical transmissions
Cell biology	Cells	Growth	Cell division
Cognitive science	Mental representations	Creation and alteration of representations	Computational procedures

enly bodies. His concept of force, however, went beyond the operation of simple machines by direct contact to include the gravitational interaction of objects at a distance from each other. In the history of science, progress has been made in many sciences by the discovery of new mechanisms, each with interacting parts affecting each other's motion and other properties. Table 7.2 displays some of the most important of these mechanisms. The sciences employ different kinds of mechanisms in their explanations, but each involves a system of parts that change as the result of interactions among them that transmit force, motion, and energy. Mechanical systems are organized hierarchically, in that mechanisms at lower levels (e.g., molecules) produce changes that take place at higher levels (e.g., cells).

Medical researchers are similarly concerned with finding mechanisms that explain the occurrence of diseases, for therapeutic as well as theoretical purposes: Understanding the mechanism that produces a disease can lead to new ideas about how the disease can be treated. In cancer research, for example, major advances were made in the 1970s and 1980s in understanding the complex of causes that lead to cancer (see chapter 1; Weinberg 1996). There are more than one hundred different kinds of cancer, but all are now thought to result from uncontrolled cell growth arising from a series of genetic mutations, first in genes for promoting growth (oncogenes) and then in genes for suppressing the tumors that are produced by uncontrolled cell growth. The mechanism of cancer production then consists of parts at two levels—cells and the

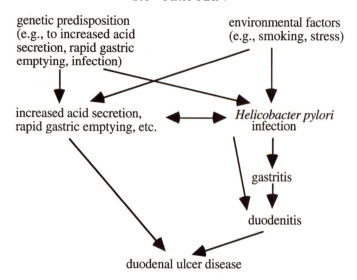

Figure 7.1. Possible mechanism of duodenal ulcer production, providing a richer causal network than that in Figure 4.1. Gastric ulcer causation is similar. Modified from Graham (1989, p. 51).

genes they contain, along with changes in cell growth produced by a series of genetic mutations. Mutations in an individual can occur for a number of causes, including heredity, viruses, and behavioral and environmental factors such as smoking, diet, and exposure to chemicals. Figure 2.7 summed up the current understanding of the mechanisms underlying cancer. This understanding is currently generating new experimental treatments based on genetic manipulations such as restoring the function of tumor suppresser genes (Bishop and Weinberg 1996).

Ulcer researchers have been concerned with the mechanism by which *H. pylori* infection produces ulcers. Figure 7.1 displays a mechanism similar to one proposed by David Graham (1989) that shows some of the interactions of heredity, environment, infection, and ulceration. Research is underway to fill in the gaps about these processes; it is looking, for example, at interactions between particular strains of *H. pylori* and the immune defenses of particular hosts.

Recent psychological research by Woo-kyoung Ahn and her colleagues has found that when ordinary people are asked to provide causes for events, they seek out information about underlying causal mechanisms as well as information about correlations (Ahn and Bailenson 1996; Ahn et al. 1995). For example, if people are asked to state the cause of John's car accident, they do not survey a range of possible factors that correlate with accidents but rather focus on the process underlying the relationship between cause and effect, such as

John's being drunk leading to erratic driving that led to the accident. Whereas causal attribution based on correlation (covariation) alone would ignore mechanisms connecting cause and effects, ordinary people are like medical researchers in that they seek mechanisms that connect cause and effect. Koslowski (1996) reports that causal reasoning in both children and adults makes good use of mechanism information as well as correlation information.

As Cheng (1997) points out, however, the emphasis on mechanism does not by itself provide an answer to the question of how people infer cause from correlation: Knowledge of mechanisms is itself knowledge of causally related events that must have somehow been previously acquired. Medical researchers inferred that bacteria cause ulcers and that smoking causes cancer when little was known about the relevant causal mechanisms. Reasoning about mechanisms can contribute to causal inference, but it is not necessary for such inference. In domains in which causal knowledge is rich, there is a kind of feedback loop in which more knowledge about causes leads to more knowledge about mechanisms, which leads to more knowledge about causes. But in less well-understood domains, correlations and the consideration of alternative causes can get causal knowledge started in the absence of much comprehension of mechanisms.

To understand how reasoning about mechanisms affects reasoning about causes, we need to consider four different situations that arise in science and ordinary life when we consider whether a factor c is a cause of an event e:

1. There is a known mechanism by which c produces e.
2. There is a plausible mechanism by which c produces e.
3. There is no known mechanism by which c produces e.
4. There is no plausible mechanism by which c produces e.

For there to be a known mechanism by which c produces e, c must be a component of or an occurrence in a system of parts that is known to interact to produce e. Only very recently has a precise mechanism by which smoking causes cancer become known: A component of cigarette smoke (Benzo[a]pyrene) was identified that produces mutations in the tumor suppresser gene *p53* (Denissenko et al. 1996). As we just saw, however, there has long been a *plausible* mechanism by which smoking causes lung cancer.

When there is a known mechanism connecting c and e, the inference that c causes e is strongly encouraged, although careful causal inference still needs to take into account information about correlations and alternative causes: A different mechanism may have produced e by an alternative cause a. For example, drunk driving often produces erratic driving that produces accidents, but even if John was drunk, his accident might have been caused by a mechanical malfunction rather than his drunkenness. Similarly, even though there is now a plausible mechanism connecting *H. pylori* infection and ulcers, we should not immediately conclude that a patient with an ulcer has the infection, since approximately twenty percent of ulcers are caused by the use of non-steroidal anti-inflammatory drugs such as aspirin. But an awareness of known and plausible mechanisms connecting c and e clearly facilitates the inference that c causes e, in a manner that is more fully spelled out later. Another way in which the plausibility of a mechanism can be judged is by analogy: If a cause and effect are similar to another cause and effect that are connected by a known mechanism, it is plausible that a similar mechanism may operate in the original case. There was a plausible mechanism by which *H. pylori* caused stomach ulcers, since other bacteria were known to produce other sores.

Sometimes causal inference from correlation can be blocked when there is no plausible mechanism connecting the event and its cause, that is, when possible mechanisms are incompatible with what is known. When Marshall and Warren first proposed that bacteria cause ulcers, the stomach was widely believed to be too acidic for bacteria to survive so there was no plausible mechanism by which bacteria could produce ulcers. Later it was found that *H. pylori* produce ammonia, which neutralizes stomach acid and thereby allows them to survive, removing the implausibility of the bacteria-ulcer mechanism. Similarly, when Alfred Wegener proposed continental drift early in this century, his theory was rejected in part because the mechanisms he proposed for continental motion were incompatible with contemporary geophysics. Only when plate tectonics was developed in the 1960s was it understood how continents can be in motion.

The two cases just mentioned are ones in which the implausibility of mechanisms was overcome, but there are many cases in which a rejection of causal relations remains appropriate. Even though there are some empirical studies that provide weak correlational evidence for extrasensory perception (ESP), it is difficult to believe that people have such powers as telepathy and telekinesis, which have properties that conflict with known physical mechanisms, such as being unaffected by spatial and temporal relations. Similarly, homeopathic medicine, which uses minute doses of drugs, violates established views concerning the amounts of substances needed to be chemically effective. A more extreme case is the theory of Velikovsky that the planet Venus once swung close to Earth and caused many historical events such as the parting of the Red Sea for Moses. Such planetary motion is totally incompatible with Newtonian mechanics, so there is no plausible mechanism by which Venus's motion could have had the claimed effect.

How can medical researchers and ordinary people combine information about mechanisms with information about correlations and alternative causes to reach conclusions about cause and effect? Recall Cheng's view (1997) that causes are theoretical entities to be inferred on the basis of correlations and alternative causes. I have argued that the justification of scientific theories, including their postulation of theoretical entities, is a matter of explanatory coherence, in which a theory is accepted because it provides a better explana-

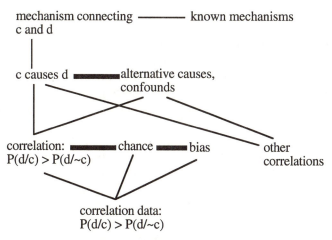

Figure 7.2. Inferring a cause *c* from correlation data about a disease *d*. That there is a correlation between *d* and *c* must be a better explanation of the observed correlation than chance or bias (or fraud). That *c* causes *d* must be a better explanation of the correlation and other correlations than alternative confounding causes. The existence of a mechanism connecting *c* and *d* provides an explanation of why *c* causes *d*. In the figure, thin lines are explanatory relations, whereas the thick lines indicate incompatibility.

tion of the evidence (see chapter 4; Thagard 1992b). Explanatory coherence of a hypothesis is a matter of both the evidence it explains and its being explained by higher level hypotheses. Charles Darwin, for example, justified the hypothesis of evolution in terms of both the biological evidence it explained and the supposition that evolution could be explained by the mechanism of natural selection. Moreover, he explicitly compared the explanatory power of his theory of evolution by natural selection with the explanatory limitations of the dominant creationist theory of the origin of species. These three factors—explaining evidence, being explained by mechanisms, and a consideration of alternative hypotheses—are precisely the same considerations that go into an evaluation of a causal hypothesis.

Figure 7.2 shows how the inference that *c* causes a disease *d* can be understood in terms of explanatory coherence. When medical researchers collect data that find a correlation between *c* and *d*, that is, a high value for $P(d/c) - P(d/{\sim}c)$, there are several possible explanations for these data. That a correlation does exist in the relevant population between *d* and *c* is one explanation for the data, but experimenters must rule out other explanations, for example, that the correlation in the data arose from chance or experimental bias. Mayo (1996) provides a thorough discussion of the use of statistical tests to rule out errors derived from chance and other factors. Another possible source of error is fraud, in which the observed correlations are based on fabricated data. Careful experimental designs involving such techniques as randomization and double blinding help rule out bias, and appropriate techniques of statistical inference tend to rule out chance, leading one to accept the hypothesis that there is a real correlation between c and d. However, before researchers can conclude that c causes d, they must have reason to believe that this hypothesis is a better explanation of the correlation than other confounding causes that might have been responsible for the correlation. Again, careful experimental design that manipulates only c or that otherwise controls for other potential causes is the key to concluding that c causes d is the best explanation of the correlation. In addition, the existence of a known or plausible mechanism for how c can produce d increases the explanatory coherence of the causal hypothesis. On the other hand, if all mechanisms that might connect c with d are incompatible with other scientific knowledge, then the hypothesis that c causes d becomes incoherent with the total body of knowledge. As Hennekens and Buring (1987) suggest, a major determinant of whether a causal hypothesis makes sense is whether it comes with a plausible underlying mechanism.

Figure 7.2 points to a synthesis of Cheng's ideas about causal powers, probabilities, and alternative causes with considerations of mechanism. Mechanisms are not a necessary condition for causal inference, but when they are known or plausible, they can enhance the explanatory coherence of a causal hypothesis. Moreover, causal hypotheses incompatible with known mechanisms are greatly reduced in explanatory coherence. Inference to causes, like inference to theoretical entities in general, depends on explanatory coherence as determined by evidence, alternative hypotheses, and higher level hypotheses.

Inference to medical causes is similar to legal inference concerning responsibility for crimes. In a murder case, for example, the acceptability of the hypothesis that someone is the murderer depends on how well that hypothesis explains the evidence, on the availability of other hypotheses to explain the evidence, and on the presence of a motive that would provide a higher level explanation of why the accused committed the murder. Motives in murder trials are like mechanisms in medical reasoning, in that they provide nonessential but coherence-enhancing explanations of a hypothesis.

This section has discussed how knowledge of mechanisms can affect inferences about causality, but it has passed over the question of how such knowledge is obtained. There are three possibilities. First, some knowledge about basic physical mechanisms may be innate, providing an infant with a head start for figuring out the world. It is possible, for example, that infants are innately equipped to infer a causal relation when one moving object bangs into another object that then starts moving. Second, some of the links in the causal chains that constitute a mechanism may be learned by induction from observed correlations as described in Cheng's Power PC model (1997). For example, we can observe the relations among pressure, temperature, and volume changes in gases and infer that they are causally connected. Third, sometimes mechanisms are abduced, that is, posited as a package of hypothetical links used to explain something observed. In cognitive science, for example, we posit computational mechanisms with various representations and processes to explain intelligent behavior. Darwin abduced the following causal chain:

variation + competition → natural selection → evolution of species

The difference between abductive and inductive inference about mechanisms is that in inductive inference the parts and processes are observed, whereas in abductive inference they are hypothesized. Knowledge about mechanisms involving theoretical (nonobservable) entities must be gained abductively, by inferring that the existence of the mechanism is the best explanation of the results of observation and experimentation. Different domains vary in the extent to which knowledge about mechanisms is innate, induced from correlations, or abductive.

DISEASE EXPLANATION AS CAUSAL NETWORK INSTANTIATION

The previous description of the interrelations of correlations, causes, and mechanisms provides the basis for an account of the nature of medical explanation. First we can eliminate a number of defective alternative accounts of explanation, including accounts in which explanation is essentially deductive, statistical, or involves single causes.

1. Explanation is not deductive. The deductive-nomological model of Hempel (1965), according to which an explanation is a deduction of a fact to be explained from universal laws, clearly does not apply to the kinds of medical explanation discussed here. Deductive explanations can be found in other fields such as physics, in which mathematical laws entail observations. But there are no general laws about the origins of ulcers and cancer. As we saw, most people with *H. pylori* do not develop ulcers, and many people without *H. pylori* do develop ulcers because of nonsteroidal anti-inflammatory drugs. Similarly, most smokers do not get lung cancer, and some nonsmokers do get lung cancer. The development of ulcers, like the development of cancer, is far too complex for general laws to provide deductive explanation.

2. Explanation is not statistical. Statistics are certainly relevant to developing medical explanations, as we saw in the contribution of the equation $P(ulcers/bacteria) - P(ulcers/no\ bacteria)$ to the conclusion that bacteria cause ulcers. But correlations themselves have no explanatory force, since they may be the result of confounding alternative causes. As we saw in Figure 7.2, the conclusion that there is a causal and hence explanatory relation between a factor and a disease depends on numerous coherence considerations, including the full range of correlations explained, the applicability of alternative causes, and the availability of a mechanism by which the factor produces the disease. A medical explanation need not show that a disease was to be expected with high probability, since the probability of getting the disease given the main cause may well be less than 0.5, as is the case for both ulcers and bacteria and lung cancer and smoking.

3. Explanation is not in terms of single causes. Although it is legitimate to see bacteria as the major causal factor in most ulcers and to see smoking as the major causal factor in most cases of lung cancer, it is simplistic to explain someone's ulcer only in terms of bacterial infection, or someone's lung cancer only in terms of smoking. As Figures 2.7 and 7.1 displayed, ulcer causation and cancer causation are complex processes that involve multiple interacting factors. Medical researchers are increasingly stressing the multifactorial nature of disease explanations. Adult-onset diabetes, for example, is now understood as arising from a complex of factors including heredity, obesity, and inactivity, all of which contribute to glucose intolerance, possibly because of a mechanism that involves a protein that reduces glucose uptake.

I propose instead that medical explanation should be thought of as *causal network instantiation*. For each disease, epidemiological studies and biological research establish a system of causal factors involved in the production of a disease. The causal network for cancer is a more elaborate version of Figure 2.7, and the causal network for ulcers is a more elaborate version of Figure 7.3, which is an elaboration of Figure 7.1. A crucial point is that the nodes in this network are connected not merely by conditional probabilities, $P(effect/cause)$, but by causal relations inferred on the basis of multiple considerations, including correlations $P(effect/cause) - P(effect/\sim cause)$, alternative causes, and mechanisms. Given this network, we explain why a given patient has a given disease by instantiating the network, that is, by specifying which factors operate in that patient. For a patient with stomach pains, a physician can start to instantiate the network in Figure 7.3 by determining whether the patient takes large quantities of nonsteroidal anti-inflammatory drugs, (e.g., because of arthritis). Different instantiation can take place on the basis of tests (e.g., endoscopy or a breath test) to determine whether the patient's stomach is infected with *H. pylori* bacteria. Some instantiation will be abductive, making hypotheses about the operation of factors that cannot be observed or tested for. The physician might make the abduction that a patient has a hereditary inclination to excess acidity, which would explain why he or she, unlike most people with *H. pylori*, has an ulcer; the hereditary abduction would be strengthened if the patient's parents and other relatives had ulcers. Similarly, to explain patients' lung cancers, we instantiate a causal network with information about their smoking, their other behaviors, their heredity, and so on. Recent work on

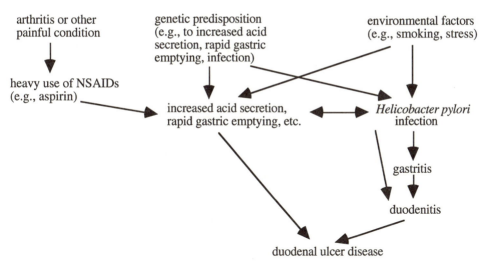

Figure 7.3. General causal network for duodenal ulcers, expanding on the network in Figure 7.1. NSAIDs are nonsteroidal anti-inflammatory drugs.

causal networks includes Glymour et al. (1987), Iwasaki and Simon (1994), Pearl (1988), and Shafer (1996).

Instantiation of a causal network such as the one in Figure 7.3 produces a kind of narrative explanation of why a person becomes sick. We can tell several possible stories about a patient, such as the following:

1. The patient became infected with *H. pylori* and developed ulcers because of a predisposition to excess acidity.

2. The patient took a lot of aspirin for arthritis and developed ulcers because of the resulting vulnerability to acidity.

But medical explanation is not just story telling, since a good medical explanation should point to all the interacting factors for which there is causal evidence and for which there is evidence of relevance to the case at hand. A narrative may be a useful device for communicating a causal network instantiation, but it is the ensemble of statistically based causal relations that is more crucial to the explanation.

Causal networks provide an explanatory schema or pattern, but they differ from the sorts of explanatory schemas and patterns proposed by others. Unlike the explanatory patterns of Kitcher (1981, 1993), causal networks are not deductive. Deductive patterns may well have applications in fields such as mathematical physics, but they are of no use in medicine, in which causal relationships are not well represented by universal laws. Unlike the explanation patterns of Schank (1986), causal networks are not simple schemas that are used to provide single causes for effects, but they instead describe complex mechanisms of multiple interacting factors. My account of medical explanation as causal network instantiation is compatible with the emphasis on mechanistic explanations by Salmon (1984) and Humphreys (1989), but it provides a fuller specification of how causal networks are constructed and applied. As already mentioned, my account of causal network installation is not compatible with interpreting the relations between factors in a causal network purely in terms of conditional probabilities.

Like the explanation of a disease in a particular patient, the explanation of why a group of people are prone to a particular disease is also a matter of causal network instantiation. People in underdeveloped countries are more likely to have gastritis than are North Americans, because poorer sanitation makes it more likely that they will acquire *H. pylori* infections that produce ulcers. Nuns are more likely to get breast cancer than are other women, because women who do not have full-term pregnancies before the age of 30 are more likely to get breast cancers, probably because of some mechanism by which pregnancy affects breast cell division. When we want to explain why a group is more likely to get a disease, we invoke the causal network for the disease and instantiate the nodes based on observations and abductions about the disease factors possessed by members of the group. Thus causal network instantiation explanations of the occurrence of both individual and group disease are structurally identical.

CONCLUSION

This chapter has shown how correlations, causes, and mechanisms all figure in the construction of causal networks that can be instantiated to provide medical explanations. The main criterion for assessing a model of disease explanation is whether it accounts for the explanatory reasoning of medical researchers and practitioners. We have seen that the causal network instantiation model of medical explanation fits well with methodological recommendations of epidemiologists such as Hennekens and Buring as well as with the practice of medical researchers working on diseases such as ulcers and lung cancer. Additional examples of the development and application of causal networks could easily be generated for other diseases such as diabetes. My account of medical explanation as causal network instantiation gains further credibility from the fact that its assumptions about the relations of correlations, causes, and mechanisms are consistent with (and provide a synthesis of) Cheng's and Ahn's psychological findings about human causal reasoning. I have not attempted to define cause in terms of explanation or explanation in terms of cause; rather, causes, mechanisms, explanations, and explanatory coherence are intertwined notions.

For some fields such as physics, the existence of universal laws and mathematical precision often makes possible explanations that are deductive. On the other hand, in fields such as economics, the lack of causal knowledge interrelating various economic factors may restrict explanations to those based on statistical associations. I expect, however, that there are many fields, such as evolutionary biology, ecology, genetics, psychology, and sociology, in which explanatory practice fits the causal network instantiation model. The possession of a feature or behavior by members of a particular species, for example, can be explained in terms of a causal network that involves mechanisms of genetics and natural selection. Similarly, the possession of a trait or behavior by a human can be understood in terms of a causal network of hereditary, environmental, and psychological factors. In psychology, as in medicine, explanation is complex and multifactorial in ways well characterized as causal network instantiation.

SUMMARY

There is much more to inferring the cause of a disease than noticing correlations with another factor. Causal reasoning requires the abductive inference that a factor has the power to produce an effect. This inference involves noticing that the effect is more probable given the factor than otherwise, but it also requires considering alternative causal factors and the plausibility of mechanisms by which the factor produces the effect. Overall, the inference that a factor is the cause of a disease is a matter of the explanatory coherence of the causal hypothesis. Disease explanations are best characterized not as deductive or statistical inferences but as instantiations of complex causal networks.

CHAPTER 8

Discovering Causes:
Scurvy, Mad Cow Disease, AIDS,
and Chronic Fatigue Syndrome

HUMANS ARE subject to many hundreds of diseases. Some of the diseases, such as cancer and epilepsy, were familiar to the ancient Greeks, whereas others such as AIDS (acquired immunodeficiency syndrome) and Lyme disease have become known only in recent decades. Solid understanding of the causes of diseases is relatively recent, stemming from such sources as the investigation of infectious diseases in the second half of the nineteenth century, the explanation of nutritional diseases in the first half of the twentieth century, and the more recent understanding of many common diseases in terms of molecular genetics (see chapter 2).

This chapter uses the history of ideas about four diseases to draw some general conclusions about why it is often so difficult to determine the causes of diseases. I first describe four overlapping stages in the development of medical understanding: disease characterization, cause specification, experimentation, and mechanism elaboration. The operation of these stages is shown in the history of four diseases (or classes of disease) that differ in the extent to which they are understood: scurvy, spongiform encephalopathies (including mad cow disease), AIDS, and chronic fatigue syndrome. Understanding of these diseases ranges from that of scurvy, which has been known to result from vitamin C deficiency since early in this century, to that of chronic fatigue syndrome, whose nature and etiology are still highly controversial. The account of causal reasoning given in chapter 7 provides a framework for understanding the difficulties of discovering the causes of disease.

STAGES OF DISEASE UNDERSTANDING

The first stage of understanding a disease is its characterization, that is, its identification as a special kind of process with its own set of symptoms that differentiate it from other diseases. This stage is not as simple as it seems, since it requires first the association of a set of characteristic symptoms and second the differentiation of the newly associated symptoms from those of other diseases. The ancient Greeks had a large category of diseases called fevers, which were considered specific diseases, not symptoms of various diseases. Many diseases have similar symptoms, so that historically there has been confusion between such diseases as smallpox and measles. Characterization of a disease, at least since the time of Hippocrates, has also involved describing the course of the disease, that is, the way its symptoms change over time.

The second stage of disease understanding is the specification of possible causes. This stage may be intermixed with the first: Sometimes two diseases are differentiated only when they are found to have different causes. Usually, however, medical practitioners have some idea about the nature of a disease before they begin to speculate about its causes. Here are three different ways in which the causes of diseases can be proposed:

> Correlation: An observed factor is found to occur with a disease, so the factor is considered to be a cause of the disease.
> Postulation: An unobserved factor is hypothesized to cause a disease.
> Biochemical analysis: Close examination of the biochemical nature of a host identifies new factors that may be a cause of the host's disease.

Historical examples of causal reasoning may involve mixtures of these three kinds of reasoning, as when the germ theory of disease led Robert Koch to postulate that a bacterium was responsible for tuberculosis and subsequently to use microscopy to identify bacteria that correlated with the disease. More examples of cause specification are provided later.

The third stage, moving from a consideration of possible causes to a conviction that the cause of a disease has been found, can be accomplished only by experimentation. Correlation, postulation, and biochemical analysis are useless unless carefully controlled experiments show that a factor is plausibly the cause of disease. The history of medicine is littered with discarded causes. To show that a correlated or hypothesized factor is the cause of a disease, it is necessary to consider other possible causes that might be responsible for the disease. The hypothesis that one factor is the cause of the disease must have more explanatory coherence than alternative hypotheses concerning other factors. A correlation between a factor and a disease might be the result of chance or other causal relations, such as there being a common cause of the factor and the disease. The four cases described subsequently illustrate the difficulty of conducting experiments that determine causality.

The fourth stage of disease understanding is the elaboration of mechanisms by which a disease is produced by its cause or causes. As earlier chapters described, many diseases are multifactorial, involving a collection of interacting causes. Mechanism elaboration usually follows experimental determination that a factor causes a disease, but an understanding of biochemical processes has sometimes been crucial in suggesting what the causes of a disease might be. Hence, these four stages of disease understanding should not be seen

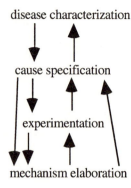

Figure 8.1. Interacting stages of disease understanding.

as discrete temporal periods but rather as four subprocesses of the process of disease understanding, as shown in Figure 8.1. For peptic ulcers, disease characterization is centuries old, but cause specification and experimentation have taken place only recently, and mechanism elaboration is still under way. To further illustrate these stages and the difficulties of discovering causes, I now briefly review the history of ideas about scurvy, spongiform encephalopathies, AIDS, and chronic fatigue syndrome.

SCURVY

In the fifteenth century, explorers from Portugal, Spain, France, and England began to make long sea voyages. By 1498, it had been noticed that sailors on these voyages often fell ill, with weakness, swollen limbs and bleeding gums (Carpenter 1986). Within a few decades, commentators had remarked that ill sailors could quickly be cured with fresh food such as oranges. But scurvy, as the disease was soon called, was not established as a nutritional deficiency until the twentieth century. Why did it take more than three hundred years to determine the cause of this disease?

Characterization of scurvy was relatively unproblematic because of the salience of the complex of symptoms that affected sea voyagers, including sores and multiple purple spots as well as the gum and limb problems just mentioned. Although it seems obvious now that the sailors suffered from a lack of vitamin C, the concept of a nutritional disease is less than a century old, dating from the discovery that beriberi was caused by a diet of polished rice (McCollum 1957). In 1622, Sir Richard Hawkins, a British sea captain who led expeditions to South America, recommended oranges and lemons as a treatment for scurvy, but he also suggested the oil of vitriol (sulfuric acid) as beneficial (Carpenter 1986, p. 15). Other recommended preventive measures included keeping the ship clean, burning tar, wearing dry clothes, exercising, and eating breakfasts of bread and diluted wine.

Sea voyages and their associated conditions were clearly responsible for the disease, but there were many unusual features of such voyages that suggested themselves as possible causes of disease. Disease specification proceeded partly in terms of correlation, as in the suggestion that the frequently damp conditions of sea travel caused sailors to become scorbutic. Another fact about sea voyages was that sailors ate a lot of salt meat, so that this was proposed as a cause of scurvy; what sailors did eat was perhaps more salient that what they did not eat. In the sixteenth through the eighteenth centuries, the dominant medical framework was still the humoral theory of Hippocrates and Galen, according to which illness is the result of a bodily imbalance among the four main fluids (humors): blood, phlegm, yellow bile, and black bile. Accordingly, Dutch physician John Echth wrote in the mid-sixteenth century that scurvy is a disease of the spleen caused by an excess of the melancholic humor, black bile.

In 1734, another Dutch physician, John Bachstrom, proposed that the absence of fresh vegetable food was the sole cause of scurvy, but his proposal was largely ignored, in part because it did not fit with general contemporary views of disease. In 1753, British surgeon James Lind published *A Treatise of the Scurvy*. Despite having performed an experiment (possibly the first controlled experiment in medical history) that found that oranges and lemons were a much better treatment for scurvy than cider, oil of vitriol, vinegar, or sea water, Lind's theory was that scurvy was the result of a cold, wet climate producing constriction of the pores that blocked perspiration. This blockage produced a concentration of humors in the body that induced scurvy, which could be treated with improvements of ships' air, acids, and lemon juice. For Lind, moisture was a more important causal factor in scurvy than diet; he argued that abstinence from vegetables and fruits could not be the primary cause of scurvy, for the ancients had not observed the disease in besieged towns where food was severely limited (Lind 1953, p. 73). The definition of scurvy in the 1933 edition of the Oxford English Dictionary states that it is "induced by exposure and by a too liberal diet of salted foods."

British naval officers such as Captain Cook took various measures against scurvy, but their mixture made it difficult to determine which ones were actually effective. One commonly used treatment was wort, a fermenting infusion of malt. By 1800, British ships routinely carried lemon or lime juice, and scurvy became much rarer, although it later arose during special situations such as the Irish potato famine of the 1850s and the long treks of arctic explorers. Lemon and lime juice did not always succeed in preventing scurvy on long voyages, probably because of the dilution and deterioration of vitamin C. Scientific developments about substances such as acids, oxygen, protein, and potassium suggested new possible causes of scurvy. The second half of the nineteenth century saw many medical breakthroughs based on the germ theory of disease, and bacterial contamination was accordingly considered as a possible cause of scurvy.

Aside from Lind's comparison of different treatments for scurvy, controlled experimentation played almost no role in the development of ideas about scurvy until the twentieth century. In 1907, two Norwegian researchers performed systematic experiments involving the causes of scurvy in guinea pigs, with results suggesting that diet was both the cause and cure of scurvy. However, a leading U.S. nutrition researcher, E. V. McCollum, rejected this view because diet did not produce scurvy in rats. At the time, it was as reasonable to take rats as a medical analog of humans as it was guinea pigs, although we now know that rats differ from humans in being able to synthesize vitamin C, so they do not require it in their diets. Experiments with monkeys showed that lemon juice provided full protection against scurvy, and attempts were made to identify the vitamin responsible for this protection. The concept of a vitamin—a factor necessary for good nutrition—was formed by Funk (1912).

In the 1920s, a Hungarian scientist, Albert Szent-Györgyi, isolated a substance he called hexuronic acid. In the 1930s, it was shown that this substance could be extracted from lemon juice and used to cure scurvy, so it was renamed ascorbic acid. Scurvy was firmly established as a nutritional disease caused by insufficient ascorbic acid. The key steps in this establishment were animal experiments showing that diet was responsible for scurvy and chemical identification of the specific substance. Later research showed that ascorbic acid is required for collagen metabolism, yielding the following mechanism:

$$\text{poor diet} \rightarrow \text{ascorbic acid deficiency} \rightarrow$$
$$\text{defective collagen biosynthesis} \rightarrow \text{scurvy.}$$

These twentieth-century breakthroughs should not obscure the previous centuries of laborious unsuccessful attempts to identify the cause of scurvy, which illustrate general difficulties of causal reasoning discussed later in this chapter.

SPONGIFORM ENCEPHALOPATHIES

Spongiform encephalopathies are members of a class of diseases found in humans and other animals. Bovine spongiform encephalopathy, also known as BSE and mad cow disease, has infected more than 100,000 British cattle since 1986, and by 1996 there was some evidence of the spread of the disease to humans. Spongiform encephalopathies are characterized by neurological degeneration that leads to progressively severe psychomotor dysfunction and death. Many researchers now believe that these diseases are caused by novel infectious proteins called prions (pronounced "pree-ons"), which were hypothesized in 1982. A review of the history of ideas about this class of diseases reveals numerous interesting aspects of medical causal reasoning.

The first disease of this class to be described was scrapie, a disease of sheep and goats that has been recognized in these animals for more than two hundred years (Collinge and Palmer 1992). A similar neurodegenerative disease in humans, marked by a rapidly progressive dementia usually followed by death within a year, was identified in the 1920s and called Creutzfeldt-Jakob disease. In the 1950s, physicians who had studied the Fore people of Papua New Guinea identified a disease the Fore called *kuru*, which was characterized by a loss of coordination, dementia, and death (Gajdusek and Zigas 1957). Initially, there was much uncertainty about the cause of the disease, which did not seem to have infectious, nutritional, or toxic origins. Early suspicion that the disease was genetic gave way, however, to the conviction that ritual cannibalism was the main cause of this disease, because of its prevalence among women and children who ate the brains of deceased relatives (Mathews et al. 1968).

The symptoms of spongiform encephalopathies are so striking that characterization of the various diseases has been unproblematic. But determination of the causes of these diseases has taken many decades, and the prion hypothesis is still somewhat controversial. In 1959, the similarity between kuru and scrapie was noticed by W. J. Hadlow (1959, 1992), a scrapie researcher who saw a museum exhibit on the Fore brain disease. He systematically laid out the similarities between the two diseases:

- Both are endemic in confined populations with a low incidence of one or two percent.
- Both have onset with no fever or other signs of illness.
- Both are almost always fatal within only a few months.
- Both involve ataxia and severe behavioral changes.
- Both are accompanied by widespread neuronal degeneration.

On the basis of the fact that scrapie had been induced experimentally in sheep, Hadlow suggested an experiment involving the induction of kuru in a laboratory primate. He could not argue analogically that the cause of kuru might specifically be identified with the cause of scrapie, which was equally unknown, but he made the important conjecture that pathogenesis of the two diseases might be similar. Daniel Gajdusek and his colleagues performed experiments showing that both kuru and Creutzfeldt-Jakob disease could be transmitted to chimpanzees, and they classified these diseases together as "transmissible spongiform encephalopathies" (Brown and Gajdusek 1991; Gajdusek, et al. 1966).

At the time, the most plausible hypothesis for the causes of these diseases concerned some kind or kinds of slow-acting virus. But Stanley Prusiner

(1982) audaciously proposed that scrapie is caused by a novel proteinaceous infectious particle, or prion. The scrapie agent had been purified from sheep brains, and investigation showed that it contained a protein required for infectivity but did not contain nucleic acids characteristic of viruses. The scrapie agent was inactivated by chemical treatments that destroyed protein but not by chemical treatments that destroyed nucleic acid. Prusiner is now sufficiently confident that spongiform encephalopathies all are caused by prions that he classes them together as *prion diseases* (Prusiner 1996; Prusiner et al. 1992). He analogically hypothesizes that other neurodegenerative diseases of humans such as Alzheimer's disease and multiple sclerosis might also be causally linked to prions (Prusiner 1982; Prusiner et al. 1992). Prusiner was awarded the 1997 Nobel Prize for medicine.

The prion hypothesis is not universally accepted, however. Some researchers believe that tests have been insufficiently sensitive to detect viral nucleic acid in the scrapie agent and that an unknown small retrovirus capable of altering host protein is the primary cause (Dal Canto 1991; Rohmer 1991). The prion hypothesis is impressive, but researchers have not been able to explain how protein particles replicate or how prions produce neurological degeneration. Moreover, viruses occur in different strains, which would explain the difficulty of transferring spongiform encephalopathies across species, whereas prions do not have multiple strains. Prusiner describes genetic differences at the level of protein production that explain why transference across species is difficult but not impossible. Work is under way to determine the mechanism by which abnormal prion protein can spread, prevent normal protein reproduction, and thereby produce defective brain development.

Acceptance of the prion hypothesis has required several important kinds of conceptual change. First, prions are a new kind of infectious agent, very different from the bacteria and viruses that have been identified as the causes of many human diseases. Second, if Prusiner's terminology is correct, the prion hypothesis has generated a new class of diseases, prion diseases, and thereby expanded the tree of infectious diseases. Third, the prion hypothesis altered the normal classification of diseases that distinguishes between infectious and hereditary diseases. Creutzfeldt-Jakob disease can develop in humans as the result of inherited defects in protein production or as the result of infection by medical procedures such as brain surgery or by eating infected beef. Thus Crentzfeldt-Jakob disease is both a hereditary and an infectious disease, collapsing the usual disease classification. A similar collapse occurs with cancer (see chapter 2), because genetic abnormalities that cause cancer can arise through inheritance, viral infection, or environmental causes. Cancer is not classed as an infectious disease, but some cancers are caused by infectious agents (e.g., Kaposi's sarcoma, which is discussed in the next section). Creutzfeldt-Jakob disease occurs sporadically and has an unknown etiology.

The apparently beef-induced cases of the disease found in 1996 seem to reflect a new variant of the disease, since they affect people much younger than those who usually get Crentzfeldt-Jakob disease.

AIDS

Between 1980 and 1995, more than 300,000 people in the United States died of AIDS, a previously unknown disease that is now the leading killer of people in that country aged twenty-five to forty-four years. Most scientists now believe that AIDS is caused by the human immunodeficiency virus (HIV). The history of medical understanding of AIDS can be divided into several periods:

1980–1984 Characterization of AIDS as a disease and the discovery of HIV.

1984–1994 Complications in and challenges to the HIV theory of AIDS.

1995–1997 Deeper understanding of the mechanisms by which HIV produces AIDS, with effective treatments using protease inhibitors.

Characterizing and explaining AIDS has been a complex and difficult project that has required the expenditure of enormous financial and human resources.

In 1980, a strange new disease was identified in gay men in Los Angeles, involving symptoms such as fever, weight loss, swollen lymph nodes, diarrhea, and thrush (Grmek 1990). Around the same time, medical personnel in New York City and San Francisco were noticing unusual occurrences of a rare cancer, Kaposi's sarcoma, in gay patients. By the end of 1981, many more cases had been identified of what was initially called GRID, for gay-related immune deficiency. Within a year, however, the disease had also been found in people other than gays, including heroin addicts and hemophiliacs, and was renamed AIDS (acquired immunodeficiency syndrome) in 1982.

The incidence of the disease strongly suggested that AIDS was caused by a bloodborne infectious agent, possibly a virus such as cytomegalovirus, which was often found in patients with Kaposi's sarcoma. Analogies with animal diseases (e.g., feline leukemia) and human infectious agents (e.g., hepatitis B virus) suggested the hypothesis that a virus was responsible for AIDS (Grmek 1990). Robert Gallo, an U.S. researcher who had discovered the first human retrovirus—HTLV-I—in 1980, suspected that the cause of AIDS was a close relative of HTLV-I (Gallo 1991, Gallo and Montagnier 1989). In 1983, separate teams of researchers led by Gallo and by Luc Montagnier in Paris identified a new retrovirus that was proclaimed as the cause of AIDS. Gallo and Montagnier (1989, p. 4) summarized the evidence:

That HIV is the cause of AIDS is by now firmly established. The evidence for causation includes the fact that HIV is a new pathogen, fulfilling the original postulate of "new disease, new agent." In addition, although the original tests found evidence of HIV infection in only a fraction of people with AIDS, newer and more sensitive methods make it possible to find such evidence in almost every individual with AIDS or pre-AIDS. Studies of blood-transfusion recipients indicate that people exposed to HIV who have no other risk factors develop AIDS. The epidemiological evidence shows that in every country studied so far AIDS has appeared only after HIV. What is more, HIV infects and kills the very T4 cells that are depleted in AIDS.

The last point concerns the mechanism by which HIV causes AIDS: HIV kills T4 cells, which are crucial to immune system operation, and thereby weakens the immune system to such an extent that infections and cancers can occur.

The discovery of HIV, however, was slow to lead to an effective treatment for AIDS, and some anomalies about the development of AIDS emerged. Researchers observed a wide variation in disease progression, with some people showing symptoms of AIDS within two or three years of infection but others showing no symptoms even after twelve years. Some scientists, such as the Berkeley virologist Peter Duesberg (1988), argued that the evidence that HIV causes AIDS was inadequate, and instead explained AIDS as the result of multiple factors such as drug use and AZT (azidothymidine). Root-Bernstein (1993) contended that AIDS is a "multifactorial, synergistic disease" that arises when the immune system is overcome by combinations of drugs, multiple infections, and allogeneic insults such as semen. Critics of the hypothesis that HIV causes AIDS complained that it had been rendered tautologous, since AIDS was diagnosed only in patients found to be HIV positive. Montagnier and Gallo began to discuss cofactors that might be required before HIV infection produced AIDS. AIDS researchers were able to rebut Duesberg's arguments by pointing to hemophiliacs and medical personnel who had acquired HIV from blood alone (Cohen 1994), but uncertainty remained about the course and treatment of the disease.

In 1995 and 1996, new research dramatically altered understanding of the causes and treatment of AIDS. HIV-1, one of the two types of HIV, was found to have at least ten distinct genetic subtypes that might vary in transmissibility (Anderson et al. 1996). Moreover, some people have genetic mutations that enable immune system cells to resist the virus. Other research refuted the view that HIV became dormant after initial infection and in fact showed that HIV produced about 10^9 virions daily (Ho et al. 1995). The immune system manages to keep HIV production in check for a long time, until the virus produces variants that can overwhelm the immune cells. This new understanding of the dynamics of HIV development coincided with the availability of a new class of antiviral drugs—protease inhibitors, which render HIV incapable of infecting new cells (Bartlett 1996). The combination of protease inhibitors with other antiviral agents has shown dramatic effects in curtailing the amount of virus in the blood and in reducing the onset and symptoms of AIDS. The effectiveness of these anti-HIV treatments strongly confirms the hypothesis that HIV causes AIDS. AIDS and peptic ulcers are similar in that both diseases involve host-strain interactions that make some people more susceptible than others, and both are best treated with combinations of drugs that overcome microbial resistance.

CHRONIC FATIGUE SYNDROME

There is now complete medical consensus concerning the causes of scurvy, and there is substantial scientific agreement concerning the causes of spongiform encephalopathies and AIDS. In sharp contrast, chronic fatigue syndrome is controversial not only with respect to its possible causes but even concerning whether it is a disease. Even the name is controversial: In the past, the disorder has been given such names as *chronic Epstein-Barr virus syndrome* and *post-viral fatigue syndrome*; in Great Britain and elsewhere, it is called *myalgic encephalomyelitis*; and some researchers and patients prefer the name *chronic fatigue/immune dysfunction syndrome* (CFIDS). Even more than the other cases I have discussed, chronic fatigue syndrome illustrates the vicissitudes of causal reasoning in medicine.

The term *chronic fatigue syndrome* was introduced in 1988 in response to reports of widespread illnesses that emerged in the United States in the mid-1980s, but retrospectively there appear to have been previous outbreaks, for example, in London in 1955 (Bell 1995, Johnson 1996, Straus 1994). Wessely (1994) argues that chronic fatigue syndrome is identical to the common nineteenth-century condition of neurasthenia. Typical symptoms of chronic fatigue syndrome include severe disabling fatigue, headache, malaise, short-term memory loss, muscle pain, trouble concentrating, joint pain, depression, abdominal pain, and many others. This multiplicity of symptoms causes great problems in characterizing and diagnosing the disorder. Bell (1995, pp. 17f) draws an analogy with AIDS:

> The parallels in the history of the recognition of AIDS as a specific disease and the recognition of CFIDS are remarkable. For years physician and health care administrators said that no illness could explain fatigue, weight loss, lymph node cancer, unusual parasitic pneumonias, and the purple spots of Kaposi's sarcoma. Because patients with AIDS were dying, it was finally and somewhat reluctantly agreed that this constellation of unusual symptoms and events was not psychosomatic. And with the discovery of the HIV virus, a theory could be put forward that explained these findings.

No similar theory has emerged to provide a unified account of why people get chronic fatigue syndrome.

In contrast to HIV tests used in diagnosing AIDS, there are no directs tests for chronic fatigue syndrome, which is diagnosed only after alternative medical and psychiatric causes of chronic fatiguing illness have been excluded (Fukuda et al. 1994). If severe fatigue has lasted more than six months and if there is no evidence for alternative causes, then chronic fatigue syndrome is diagnosed if four or more of the following eight symptoms are present: impaired memory or concentration, sore throat, tender cervical or auxiliary lymph nodes, muscle pain, multijoint pain, new headaches, unrefreshing sleep, and postexertion malaise.

Since the 1980s outbreak, researchers have looked for a viral cause of chronic fatigue syndrome. An early proposal that a retrovirus similar to HTLV-II is responsible was not confirmed, and numerous hypotheses about the nature of chronic fatigue syndrome are still under debate:

1. Chronic fatigue syndrome is not a disease or even a syndrome (i.e., a recurring pattern of symptoms) but an ill-formed category that covers fatigue resulting from many other medical and psychiatric conditions, such as multiple sclerosis.

2. Chronic fatigue syndrome is a psychiatric illness primarily due to depression or neurosis.

3. Chronic fatigue syndrome is caused by an undiscovered virus that overactivates the immune system, producing excessive amounts of cytokines such as interferon that cause multiple symptoms (Bell 1995).

4. Chronic fatigue syndrome is an immune system disorder that can be triggered by many different infectious agents, including enteroviruses, the Epstein-Barr virus, and human herpesvirus-6 (Fekety 1994).

Defenders of the reality of chronic fatigue syndrome argue against the first hypothesis by pointing to the commonality of symptoms among people with chronic fatigue in geographically identifiable outbreaks such as that in Lake Tahoe in 1985. The second hypothesis is challenged by pointing out that depression is found in only sixty percent of chronic fatigue syndrome patients and is characterized by frustration at not being able to perform normal activities rather than by despair and apathy.

It is currently impossible to choose between the third and fourth hypotheses, neither of which has much evidential support. If chronic fatigue syndrome is indeed like AIDS, a novel virus will be identified that can produce the appropriate range of symptoms, and the third hypothesis will meet with rapid acceptance. On the other hand, acceptance of the fourth hypothesis will require substantial advances in knowledge concerning the mechanisms of infection and immune system reaction, displaying a common pathway from infection to fatigue. Psychiatric aspects such as depression and stress may well turn out to be cofactors influencing this pathway.

To someone seeking medical simplicity, chronic fatigue syndrome is a condition with too many names, too many symptoms, and too many possible causes. Perhaps it will fade into medical history, as neurasthenia did in the nineteenth century. A more medically satisfying outcome will require research breakthroughs concerning the causes and mechanisms of chronic fatigue syndrome.

COMPLEXITIES OF CAUSAL INFERENCE

The diseases whose history I have sketched illustrate the difficulties of determining the causes of disease, which can be framed in terms of the model of causal inference proposed in chapter 7. The inference that a factor is a cause of a disease is based on explanatory coherence: We can infer that the factor causes the disease if this hypothesis is part of the best explanation of the full range of evidence. Collecting data that the factor and the disease are positively correlated (i.e., that the probability of the disease given the factor is greater than the probability of disease without the factor) does not suffice to show that the factor causes the disease. The correlation in the data may be due to chance or bias in data collection, and we must be able to infer that a genuine correlation is the best explanation of the observed correlation. Even if the correlation is genuine, it may not indicate a causal relation, since various alternative causes may be responsible for the correlation. That the factor causes the disease must be a better explanation of the correlation between the factor and the diseases than the assertion that some other cause is responsible for both the factor and the disease. Confidence that the factor causes the disease is increased if there is a familiar mechanism that explains why or how the factor causes the disease (see Figure 7.2).

Disease Characterization

Before causal inference can get underway, there needs to be a disease to be explained. This is problematic, however, in cases such as AIDS and chronic fatigue syndrome, in which many different symptoms are involved. Historically, it has not been easy to demarcate symptoms, syndromes, and diseases. AIDS was initially identified as a syndrome but has been recognized as a disease since the causal factor HIV was identified as common to all cases. Chronic fatigue syndrome will likely remain just that—a syndrome—until the causes and mechanisms are better understood. Many other diseases, however, such as scurvy and kuru have sufficiently distinct symptomologies that they could be characterized as diseases long before their etiologies are understood. But for some diseases, indeterminacy of symptoms is an impediment to the development of causal understanding. Additional impediments fall into three classes: identifying possible causes, experimentally demonstrating causality, and establishing mechanisms.

Cause Identification

Identifying possible causes of a disease can be difficult for several reasons. First, as in the history of scurvy, there can be too many possible causes to sort out. Sea voyages on which sailors contracted scurvy were as strongly associated with damp air as with bad diet, and even within the diet there were factors such as salty meat that were more salient that the absence of fresh fruits and vegetables. AIDS was found to correlate with many factors, including both sexual activity and drug use, making it difficult to determine which correlations were causally significant.

A second impediment to identifying causally relevant correlates of diseases can be background causal beliefs. In the first two centuries of the investigation of scurvy, there was no natural place for dietary deficiency in the humoral theory of disease or in the germ theory of disease that successively dominated medical thinking. Similarly, recognition that beriberi is a nutritional disease was impeded by attempts to find a microbial cause. The prion hypothesis was initially suspect because of the belief that infectious agents require DNA or RNA for replication. Convictions that chronic fatigue syndrome is a psychiatric disorder discourage the search for a responsible causal agent. Similarly, when the theory that peptic ulcers are caused by bacteria was first proposed in 1983, it was greeted with skepticism in part because of the belief that the stomach's acidity produces a sterile environment (see chapter 4). The delay of almost two hundred years from the observation of bacteria by Antonie van Leeuwenhoek to the development of the germ theory of disease was partly the result of the influence of the humoral theory.

A third difficulty in identifying possible causes of diseases is that many causes are not directly observable. Bacteria became observable only with the invention of the optical microscope, and viruses became observable only with the invention of the electron microscope (see chapter 5). Even with modern technology, bacteria and viruses are not always easy to identify, as is shown by discoveries in only the past few decades of new kinds of bacteria that are responsible for peptic ulcers, Lyme disease, and Legionnaire's disease, as well as the discoveries of medically important viruses such as HIV. Correlating a disease with a factor is obviously impeded by an inability to observe the factor. The difficulty is even greater when the cause is not a microbe but rather a complex biochemical process that involves interactions of genes, proteins, and environmental conditions (see chapter 2).

Experimentation

The three difficulties just described concern the search for possible causes to correlate with diseases. Finding that a factor is correlated with a disease obviously does not show it to be a cause of the disease, for the factor may be a result of the real cause of the disease or may be only accidentally related. The best way to show that correlation indicates causation is to conduct controlled experiments that rule out other causal factors. In medicine, however, such experiments are not always possible. Sailors could not go on voyages without damp air, and researchers could not ethically inject patients with HIV to see if they develop AIDS. Hence the first difficulty in experimentally demonstrating the causes of diseases is that fully controlled experiments are often not practicable or ethical.

The second difficulty in experimentally showing the causes of diseases is that animal models may be unavailable or misleading. Animal models often provide a means of conducting controlled experiments, but they are not always available or accurate. Demonstration that scurvy is caused by nutritional deficiency benefited from experiments with guinea pigs, but experiments with rats were misleading. Gajdusek's experiments with chimpanzees were crucial in establishing that kuru and Creutzfeldt-Jakob disease are caused by a transmissible agent, but there appear to be differences between the prions involved in diseases in different animals. These differences make some inferences problematic, for example, concerning how likely it is that bovine spongiform encephalopathy will spread to humans. Animals models for HIV infection have been difficult to establish and interpret, because the virus behaves differently in other animals than it behaves in humans. Chronic fatigue syndrome is not even close to having any kind of animal model.

The third difficulty in experimentally showing disease causality arises from the complexity of many disease processes. Some diseases, such as spongiform encephalopathies and AIDS, may take years to develop, making it difficult to determine the effects of different kinds of experimental manipulations. Moreover, many diseases are multifactorial, with many contributing causes. Infectious diseases not only are the result of the invasion of the host by a microbe but also may depend on various features of the host, such as immune system status, and on interactions between the strains of the microbe and the host. When a disease has interacting causes, it can be difficult to isolate experimentally a particular factor as a major cause. Some sailors on long voyages did not get scurvy; only a few British beef eaters have so far developed the new variant of Creutzfeldt-Jakob disease; and exposure to HIV does not always produce infection and AIDS. There are some diseases (e.g., genetic conditions such as Huntington's disease) for which we can unambiguously establish a unitary cause-disease relation, but most human diseases involve more complicated processes that have multiple causes.

Mechanism Elaboration

In addition to the three difficulties of identifying possible causes and the three difficulties of experimentally demonstrating causality, there is a remaining difficulty concerning the description of mechanisms. Our confidence that a factor really is a major cause of a disease is greatly increased if we can describe in detail the biochemical process by which the cause produces the disease and its symptoms. By and large, such understanding has become possible only in the last few decades through the rapid developments in molecular biology. We can say that vitamin C deficiency causes bleeding gums and other problems because it is needed for collagen metabolism. Prion researchers are increasingly understanding how defects in proteins can lead to brain disorders. The molecular genetics of HIV are sufficiently well understood that effective antiviral drugs such as protease inhibitors have been produced. Unfortunately, there are many conditions and diseases, ranging from chronic fatigue syndrome to atherosclerosis to arthritis, for which the causal mechanisms are poorly understood.

The difficulties of determining causes that occur at the different stages of disease understanding are summarized in Table 8.1. It is impressive that, despite these difficulties in determining the causes of diseases, modern medicine has made remarkable progress. It took more than three hundred years to identify vitamin C deficiency as the crucial factor in scurvy, and sixty years to identify prions as the cause of Creutzfeldt-Jakob disease. Strikingly, the period from the characterization of AIDS to the identification of HIV as the plausible cause of AIDS was only three years. Progress on chronic fatigue syndrome has not been so impressive, but serious investigation using the full resources of epidemiology and molecular medicine has been underway only since 1988. The scientific sophistication of medical research has expanded dramatically since the mid-nineteenth century, with improved theories, technologies, and experimental methodologies. Randomized controlled studies became the accepted norm for medical research only in the second half of the twentieth century (see chapter 12).

Initially, it seems amazing that the cause of peptic ulcers was discovered only in the 1980s, but the four diseases discussed in this chapter show that the path to uncovering disease causality is often difficult. The 1980s investigation of peptic ulcers did not have the difficulty found with AIDS and chronic fatigue syndrome of having a confusing complex of symptoms, but all the other

TABLE 8.1

Difficulties of Discovering Causes in Four Stages of Disease Understanding

Disease characterization
 1. A condition may have diverse symptoms and be hard to recognize as a disease.

Cause specification
 2. A disease may be correlated with many possible causes.
 3. Background theories may impede the recognition of plausible causes.
 4. Causes of diseases may be nonobservable.

Experimentation
 5. Controlled experiments in humans may be impracticable or unethical.
 6. Animal models may be unavailable or misleading.
 7. Multifactorial diseases involve complex interactions.

Mechanism elaboration
 8. Causal mechanisms may be difficult to discover and describe.

seven difficulties listed in Table 8.1 apply. And disease characterization *is* a problem for dyspepsia, which is sometimes caused by *H. pylori*; (see chapter 12).

Discovering and establishing causal factors for diseases is a complex cognitive task that requires great ingenuity in identifying possible causes and in performing controlled experiments to rule out alternative causes. My account in this chapter of scurvy, spongiform encephalopathies, AIDS, and chronic fatigue syndrome has been much briefer than my description of the bacterial theory of ulcers, and it has ignored physical and social processes in favor of cognitive ones. But it has served to display further the complexities of causal reasoning in medicine.

SUMMARY

Understanding a disease requires characterizing its symptoms, specifying possible causes, determining actual causes experimentally, and elaborating the mechanism by which the cause produces the disease. It took four hundred years for the causes of scurvy to be understood, because of the multiplicity of possible causes and the interference of the humoral and germ theories of disease. An understanding of the spongiform encephalopathies was delayed for decades by difficulties in identifying the highly unusual infectious agent that is responsible for the class of diseases. The cause of AIDS was found within a few years of the characterization of the disease but remained controversial until more was learned about the behavior and variants of the

HIV virus. Chronic fatigue syndrome is a difficult subject for scientific investigation, because its symptoms are variable and no causal agent has been identified. Determining the causes of diseases is a complex process that can be hindered by serious impediments to discovery and experimentation (see Table 8.1).

CHAPTER 9

Medical Analogies

CAUSAL REASONING based on explanatory coherence is a major part of medical thinking, but other cognitive processes are also important to understanding the development and application of medical knowledge. One such process is analogy, in which a previously solved problem serves as a source for solving a new target problem. I have already briefly mentioned some analogies that have been important in medical cases, such as the analogies between disease and fermentation (see chapter 2), between ulcers and other infectious diseases (see chapter 3), and between kuru and scrapie (see chapter 7). This chapter describes in more detail the purposes served by medical analogies (i.e., why they are used) and the different cognitive processes that support those purposes (i.e., how they are used). Historical and contemporary examples illustrate the theoretical, experimental, diagnostic, therapeutic, technological, and educational value of medical analogies. Four models of analogical transfer illuminate how analogies are used in these cases.

MODELS OF ANALOGICAL TRANSFER

The widespread use of analogies in cognition, including scientific reasoning, has been well documented (e.g., Biela 1991; Gentner et al. 1997; Holyoak and Thagard 1995; Leatherdale 1974). Analogical transfer, in which people use a source problem to provide a solution to a target problem, can take place in at least four different ways. The model of analogical transfer most commonly discussed in cognitive science works as follows. First, someone attempts to solve a target problem and then remembers or is given a similar source problem for which a solution is known. The target problem is then solved by adapting the solution to the source problem to provide a solution to the target. Many psychological experiments have followed this pattern (e.g., Gick and Holyoak 1980). And many computational models of analogical problem solving, including most work on case-based reasoning, also fit this pattern (e.g., Kolodner 1993). Accordingly, I use the term *standard model* for this pattern of retrieving a source to solve a target problem.

There are, however, other ways in which people use analogies to solve problems. In the standard model, the target problem serves as a direct retrieval cue for the source problem, but retrieval can also take place more indirectly using a schema that is abstracted from the target problem. According to the *schema model*, an attempt to solve a target problem produces an abstract schema that then serves as a powerful retrieval cue for finding a source problem that provides a solution to the target problem. Although the abstraction may directly suggest a solution to the target problem, it may less directly suggest a solution by producing recall of a particular case that is sufficiently similar to the target to serve as the source of a solution. Darden (1983) discusses analogies in terms of shared abstractions.

In both the standard and schema models, the thinker starts with a target problem and retrieves a source, but there are important cases in which the act of reminding works in the opposite direction. These cases are ones in which an attempt to solve a target problem has failed, and the problem solver leaves it aside. Later, however, the problem solver serendipitously encounters a solved problem that can serve as a potential source, and this new source prompts recall of the unsolved target problem. Instead of the target providing a retrieval cue for the source, the source provides a retrieval cue for the target. The *serendipity model* refers to a pattern of analogical transfer in which a target problem is recalled and solved using a source accidentally encountered after initial solutions fail (cf. Langley and Jones 1988). Darwin's discovery of the theory of evolution by natural selection fits well the serendipity model: Darwin had long wondered about how biological evolution occurs, he found a solution only when he read Malthus and realized that Malthus's ideas about human population growth could be adapted to provide an explanation of species evolution in terms of the struggle for existence.

In all three models so far described, the source problem exists independently of the target problem. But there are rich analogies in which the source problem is constructed to provide a solution to the target problem. Nersessian (1992) describes how Maxwell generated a theoretical explanation of electromagnetism by constructing a mechanical analog. He did not understand electromagnetism in terms of any known mechanical system but instead concocted a new mechanical system that suggested the equations that he was then able to apply to electromagnetism. I use the term *generation model* for analogical transfer that takes place when a target problem is solved by analogy with a specially constructed source problem. The process of generation of a source analogy is roughly this:

1. Start with a target problem.
2. Retrieve or encounter a very approximate analog.
3. Fill out the approximate analog by looking at the target and identifying aspects of the constructed analog that need identification.
4. Transfer from the newly constructed source to the target.

The standard, schema, serendipity, and generation models are complementary accounts of analogical transfer rather than competitors (Figure 9.1). Dif-

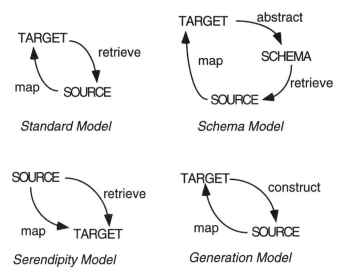

Figure 9.1. Models of analogical transfer.

ferent episodes of human analogical problem solving employ all four of the reasoning strategies that the models describe. In particular, there are important medical analogies that instantiate each of these models.

THEORETICAL ANALOGIES

Theoretical analogies are those that are important in the development and justification of explanatory hypotheses. Important theoretical analogies in physics include the comparison of sound with water waves and of light waves with sound waves. Biology has also employed analogies that have contributed to theoretical development, such as Darwin's analogy between natural and artificial selection. Theoretical analogies have been equally important in the history of medicine, from the Hippocratics to the development of the germ theory of disease and beyond. The ancient Greeks explained health in terms of a balance of the various qualities that constituted the body, using a term for balance, *isonomia*, that also connoted equality of political rights (Temkin 1977, p. 272). The great seventeenth-century physician Thomas Sydenham conceived of diseases as akin to biological species, maintaining that just as characteristics of a plant species are extended to every individual so the characteristics of a disease apply to every individual who has it (Bynum 1993, p. 341).

In 1847, a physician in Vienna, Ignaz Semmelweiss, used a serendipitous analogy to form a hypothesis concerning the cause of childbed fever that was common among women who had been examined by medical students (Sinclair

1909). His colleague Kolletschka cut his finger during an autopsy and became very sick with the same symptoms as women with childbed fever. Semmelweiss hypothesized that Kolletschka had become ill because of contamination from a cadaver, and he proposed analogously that women were being made ill by medical students who had been performing autopsies.

The most important theoretical analogy in the history of medicine was used by Louis Pasteur and Joseph Lister in the development of the germ theory of disease. In the 1850s and 1860s, they realized that just as fermentation is caused by yeast and bacteria, so diseases may also be caused by microorganisms. Pasteur's ideas about infection moved from using microorganisms to explain why milk, beer, and wine ferment to proposing similar explanations of diseases in silkworms to explaining human diseases such as rabies in terms of germs. Pasteur wrote concerning his work on fermentation:

> What meditations are induced by those results! It is impossible not to observe that, the further we penetrate into the experimental study of germs, the more we perceive sudden lights and clear ideas on the knowledge of the causes of contagious diseases! Is it not worthy of attention that, in that Arbois vineyard (and it would be true of the million *hectares* of vineyards of all the countries in the world), there should not have been, at the time I made the aforesaid experiments, one single particle of earth which would not have been capable of provoking fermentation by a grape yeast, and that, on the other hand, the earth of the glass houses I have mentioned should have been powerless to fulfill that office? And why? Because, at the given moment, I covered that earth with some glass. The death, if I may so express it, of a bunch of grapes, thrown at that time on any vineyard, would infallibly have occurred through the *saccharomyces* parasites of which I speak; that kind of death would have been impossible, on the contrary, on the little space enclosed by my glass houses. Those few cubic yards of air, those few square yards of soil, were there, in the midst of a universal possible contagion, and they were safe from it. . . . Is it not permissible to believe, by analogy, that a day will come when easily applied preventive measures will arrest those scourges which suddenly desolate and terrify populations; such as the fearful disease (yellow fever) which has recently invaded Senegal and the valley of the Mississippi, or that other (bubonic plague), yet more terrible perhaps, which has ravaged the banks of the Volga? (translated in Vallery-Radot 1926, pp. 287–288; for the original, see Pasteur 1922, Vol. 2, p. 547).

Pasteur's theoretical analogy had the following structure :

Fermentation is caused by germs.
Disease is like fermentation.
Disease may therefore also be caused by germs.

As far as one can tell from the historical record, the development of Pasteur's ideas appears to fit with the standard model of analogical transfer. In working on silkworms, he was able to draw on his previous work on fermentation, and in working on human diseases, he drew on the ideas and techniques that had been useful with silkworms. The previously understood problems of fermentation and silkworm diseases provided sources for analogical solution of the subsequent target problem of human disease.

A similar theoretical analogy was also important in the development of modern surgery. Before the 1860s, many surgical patients suffered serious infections, which were not explained until the British surgeon Lister realized the significance of Pasteur's ideas about fermentation and recognized that germs in the air can cause infection of wounds, just as they cause fermentation. He wrote in 1867:

> Turning now to the question how the atmosphere produces decomposition of organic substances, we find that a flood of light has been thrown upon this most important subject by the philosophic researches of M. Pasteur, who has demonstrated by thoroughly convincing evidence that it is not to its oxygen or to any of its gaseous constituents that the air owes this property, but to the minute particles suspended in it, which are the germs of various low forms of life, long since revealed by the microscope, and regarded as merely accidental concomitants to putrescence, but now shown by Pasteur to be its essential cause, resolving the complex organic compounds into substances of simpler chemical constitution, just as the yeast plant converts sugar into alcohol and carbonic acid. . . . Applying these principles to the treatment of compound fracture, bearing in mind that it is from the vitality of the atmospheric particles that all mischief arises, it appears that all that is requisite is to dress the wound with some material capable of killing those septic germs, provided that any substance can be found reliable for this purpose, yet not too potent as a caustic. (reprinted in Brock 1961, p. 84)

The structure of Lister's reasoning was as follows:

Fermentation is caused by germs.
Putrefaction (infection) following surgery is like fermentation.
Putrefaction may therefore be caused by germs.

This analogical transfer does not fit the standard model, since Lister must have worried about the problem of wound infection for many years before reading Pasteur's work on fermentation, which reminded him of the pre-existing wound target problem. In this case, the source problem (fermentation) prompted retrieval of the target problem (infection), so it best fits the serendipity model of analogical transfer.

The analogy between fermentation and infection was a remote one, since on the face of it there is little apparent similarity between grapes becoming alcoholic and wounds becoming infected. Closer analogies are ubiquitous in medical research, which relies heavily on the use of animal models to determine the causes of disease. For example, Robert Koch determined that tuberculosis is caused by a bacterium by performing experiments on guinea pigs. He showed that injecting guinea pigs with bacteria taken from other guinea pigs with tuberculosis induced tuberculosis in them. Obviously, it would be unethical to induce tuberculosis in humans in this way and therefore impossible to do a controlled experiment of tuberculosis in humans. Koch used animals to *generate* an analog to human disease (Brock 1988). This is not a case of analogical transfer by reminding or serendipity but rather of constructing an animal analog that can then be used to make inferences about human diseases. The structure of the analogical transfer in these cases is roughly as follows:

> We want to know the causes of a disease in humans.
> Animals (e.g., guinea pigs) have the same (or similar) disease.
> In animals, the disease is caused by X.
> The human disease may therefore also be caused by something like X.

The constructive nature of animal analogies is even more evident when new animal strains are created to provide models for human diseases. Biologists, for example, have used genetic engineering to create a strain of mouse that develops Alzheimer's disease. Because the mouse develops the types of plaques on the brain that are found in humans with Alzheimer's and also suffers memory problems, it can be used in experiments that are aimed at determining the causes of and possible treatments for Alzheimer's disease. Analogies based on animal models are also important for therapeutic purposes (see later). Sometimes, animal models are arrived at serendipitously, as when researchers who set out to genetically engineer rats as a model of human arthritis discovered that they had created a model of ulcerative colitis. As I mentioned in chapter 3, early attempts to use pigs as an animal model for *H. pylori* infection failed, but later efforts with bacteria-free piglets were more successful. Animal experimentation has nevertheless played a very minor role in development of the bacterial theory of ulcers.

Animal analogies were important in the development of ideas about nutritional deficiency diseases. Understanding of beriberi was greatly advanced when a similar disease was found in chickens that had been fed polished rice, and chapter 8 described how guinea pigs served as a valuable animal model for human scurvy. Funk (1912), having isolated what he thought was the vitamin needed to prevent beriberi, analogically suggested methods for isolating the vitamin that he conjectured was similarly responsible for scurvy. Moreover, on the basis of similarities with beriberi and scurvy, he correctly speculated that pellagra and rickets are also deficiency diseases.

Critics of animal experimentation have raised doubts about the ability of such models to provide explanations of human diseases (LaFollette and Shanks 1995). Animal models often break down because of physiological differences between humans and the animals used, which also lead to differences in causality and treatment effectiveness. Treatments that are effective in animals or in the test tube often do not work on humans. Analogical reasoning is frequently a risky kind of inference, but Holyoak and Thagard (1995) describe various steps that can be taken to improve the quality of analogical reasoning. We urged analogists to use *system mappings*, ones based on deep similarities of causal relations rather than on superficial similarities. When animal experimentation uses animals whose physical processes are known to be similar to those of humans, there can be a system mapping based on the existence of similar causal mechanisms. We also urged analogists to use multiple analogies, that is, to consider the relevance of various possible source analogs for the case at hand. Well-informed medical researchers look at various possible animal models for a human disease and base their experimental conclusions on deep causal similarities between the animals and humans. Under these conditions, animal models provide generated theoretical analogies that are at least suggestive about the causes of diseases in humans.

A related issue is the value of animal models of human thinking. On the one hand, the assumption of behaviorist psychologists that the rat could serve as a full model of human learning grossly underestimated the cognitive differences between humans and rats. On the other hand, neuroscientific research has found important similarities in humans and other animals with respect to visual and emotional systems.

Medical thinking about some human diseases has also been aided by analogies with similar diseases. Researchers on tuberculosis made comparisons with similar infectious diseases such as smallpox and syphilis, and researchers on yellow fever made comparisons with malaria. These analogies are relatively close ones that generally fit the standard model of analogical transfer, as with Robert Gallo's attempt to find a virus that causes AIDS that is analogous to those viruses with which he was already familiar (see chapter 8). In turn, AIDS has served as a suggestive analogy for some investigators of chronic fatigue syndrome. Recent speculations that atherosclerotic coronary heart disease might be caused by an infection of *Chlamydia pneumoniae* are defended by comparison with the discovery of a bacterial cause for another inflammatory/degenerative disease, peptic ulcers (Muhlestein 1997).

As I mentioned in chapter 8, analogies contributed to the development of ideas about kuru. Hadlow (1959) noticed similarities between the sheep disease scrapie and the New Guinea disease kuru and suggested experiments to determine if the latter was also transmissible. Research on these brain diseases led to Stanley Prusiner's (1982) hypothesis concerning a novel infectious agent called prions, which he analogically suggested might also be responsible for other diseases, such as Alzheimer's. According to Rhodes (1997, p. 101), two of the anthropologists who first made the connection between kuru and cannibalism did so because of a strange analogy. Shirley Lindenbaum and Robert Glasse left Australia for New Guinea in 1961 and in 1962 read a *Time* magazine story that a scientist had trained flatworms to find their way through a maze, chopped them up, and fed them to other flatworms that then got through the maze. This result (which has since been discredited) provided the anthropologists with a rough model to suggest that the brain problems of the Fore people might be caused by their cannibalism.

I have included in this section only analogies that are important in the development and justification of explanatory hypotheses. Explanatory analogies whose function is primarily expository are discussed in the later section on educational analogies. Some philosophers and scientists are skeptical that analogy can play any role in justifying hypotheses; see Thagard (1992b) for a defense of the relevance of analogy to justification as well as discovery. Analogy is a contributor to explanatory coherence, and analogical mapping and retrieval can be understood computationally as coherence problems (Holyoak and Thagard 1995; Thagard and Verbeurgt 1998).

EXPERIMENTAL ANALOGIES

To establish a medical hypothesis, controlled experiments are needed to distinguish causation from mere correlations. Epidemiologists have established numerous standards for designing experiments that address the causes of diseases. Because of the complexity of experimentation, however, it is unlikely that medical researchers design their experiments from scratch. Experiments can be designed via an application of the standard model of analogical transfer, when a researcher remembers a previous experiment that suggests how to do the desired new experiment. Dunbar (1995, 1997) describes the frequent use of analogies in the design of experiments in molecular biology, and Kettler and Darden (1993) describe a program that uses analogy to help design protein sequencing experiments.

Experimental analogies have the following structure:

We need to do an experiment to accomplish X.
A previous experiment accomplished Y, a task similar to X.
We can therefore do a modification of the previous experiment.

It is also possible that analogical transfer in experimental design could fit the serendipity model. A researcher might wonder how to design an experiment to test a hypothesis and then encounter a paper describing an experimental procedure that tests a similar hypothesis. The researcher could then design a similar experiment.

DIAGNOSTIC ANALOGIES

Medical research aims at discovering the causes of diseases, but the reasoning task facing most physicians consists of diagnosing the presence of disease in individual patients. The physician needs to decide what disease or complex of diseases provides the best explanation of the patient's symptoms. This task often does not involve analogy. In straightforward cases, it can be almost deductive: If the patient has symptoms S1, S2, and S3, then it is almost certain that the patient has the disease D. In more complex cases, the reasoning is abductive, with the physician having to select, from a variety of diseases that would explain the patient's symptoms, a diagnosis that fits best with what is known.

Sometimes, however, a diagnosis problem does not admit a simple deductive or abductive solution, and analogies may then be useful. The general structure of diagnostic analogies is as follows:

The patient P has the unusual set of symptoms, S1, S2, and S3.
Another patient with similar symptoms had a disease D.
The patient P may therefore also have the disease D.

Koton (1988) describes a case-based–reasoning program that produces causal explanations of a heart patient's symptoms by retrieving examples of similar patients.

THERAPEUTIC ANALOGIES

In addition to performing the task of diagnosis, medical reasoners want to be able to treat patients in ways that cure their diseases or at least reduce their symptoms. Berlinger (1996) describes a dramatic case of a baby born with a cystic cygroma that made it very difficult to breathe. When the baby stopped breathing, it became crucial to insert a tube in the baby's airway, but a cluster of yellow cysts hid the airway so that it was not clear where to insert the tube. Berlinger fortunately remembered a previous case in which an emergency technician had inserted a breathing tube to save the life of a snowmobiler with a severed windpipe by sticking the tube where bloody bubbles indicated the airway. Analogously, Berlinger pushed down on the baby's chest to push air out through the cysts, generating saliva bubbles that he could use as a guide for insertion of the breathing tube. This therapeutic analogy fits the standard model of analogical transfer, with the physician retrieving a source problem (the snowmobiler's inability to breathe) to solve the target problem (the baby's inability to breathe). There are undoubtedly more prosaic cases in which physicians prescribe treatments because they worked previously with the same or similar patients.

Therapeutic analogies can also be based on similarities between diseases. Greenberg and Root (1995) describe a case in which a physician was unable to diagnose a particular disease or diseases in a patient with a complex set of symptoms. However, because the patient's symptoms were similar to those of patients with identified diseases who had been successfully treated, the physician recommended a similar treatment. This case fits the standard model of analogical transfer.

At a more general level, therapeutic analogies can be drawn from animal models used in experiments to determine the effectiveness of treatments for diseases. The general structure of these analogies is as follows:

We want to know the medical effects of a treatment in humans.
Animals (e.g., guinea pigs) are similar to humans.
We can therefore try the treatment first in animals.
We can then transfer the conclusions (positive or negative) back to humans.

As with the animal model analogies described in the previous section on theoretical analogies, these analogies fit the generative model of transfer, and the value of the animal therapeutic analogies depends on the relational similarity of the relevant causal processes in animals and humans.

Finally, here is an analogy used to suggest early and aggressive treatment of HIV infections (Ho et al. 1995, p. 126):

The CD4 lymphocyte depletion seen in advanced HIV-1 infection may be likened to a sink containing a low water level, with the tap and drain both equally wide open. As the regenerative capacity of the immune system is not infinite, it is not difficult to see why the sink eventually empties. It is also evident from this analogy that our primary strategy to reverse the immunodeficiency ought to be to target virally mediated destruction (plug the drain) rather than to emphasize lymphocyte reconstitution (put in a second tap).

TECHNOLOGICAL ANALOGIES

Medicine requires many technologies for the diagnosis, treatment, and prevention of disease. A technological analogy is one in which transfer produces a new medical tool. I discuss three examples: Lister's treatment of wounds, the invention of the stethoscope, and the invention of the polymerase chain reaction.

Lister's analogy between fermentation and putrefaction suggested a means of preventing infection. He recalled that carbolic acid had been used in Carlisle on sewage to prevent odor and diseases in cattle that fed on the pastures irrigated from the refuse material; he accordingly began to use carbolic acid to sterilize wounds, which dramatically decreased the infection rate. This analogical transfer fits the standard model. Having inferred from Pasteur's work that germs from the air might cause putrefaction, he generated a new solution to the target problem of how to prevent germs from infecting wounds. This problem reminded him of the use of carbolic acid in Carlisle, which he then applied successfully (if not pleasantly) to surgery.

Earlier in the nineteenth century, a French physician had used analogy in the invention of the most widely used piece of medical technology, the stethoscope. There are two different historical accounts of this discovery, alternatively fitting the schema and serendipity models of analogical transfer. Here is Théophile Laennec's (1962, pp. 284–285) own description in 1819 of how he invented the stethoscope:

> In 1816, I was consulted by a young woman labouring under general symptoms of diseased heart, and in whose case percussion and the application of the hand were of little avail on account of the great degree of fatness. The other method just mentioned [application of the ear to the chest] being rendered inadmissible by the age and sex of the patient, I happened to recollect a simple and well-known fact in acoustics, and fancied, at the same time, that it might be turned to some use on the present occasion. The fact I allude to is the augmented impression of sound when conveyed through certain solid bodies,—as when we hear the scratch of a pin at one end of a piece of wood, on applying our ear to the other. Immediately, on this suggestion, I rolled a quire of paper into a sort of cylinder and applied it to one end of the region of the heart and the other to my ear, and was not a little surprised and pleased, to find that I could thereby perceive the action of the heart in a manner much more clear and distinct than I had ever been able to do by the immediate application of the ear.

This account fits with the schema model of analogical transfer: Laennec solved the target problem of how to listen to the woman's heart by abstracting it into a general acoustic problem that reminded him of pin scratching a piece of wood. The wood then served as a source that suggested the use of a rolled-up piece of paper to listen to the woman's heart. In Laennec's account, a general acoustic fact provided the retrieval cue for finding a source problem that could be used to produce a solution to the target problem.

A different account has, however, found its way into the historical record, owing to Laennec's friend Lejumeau de Kergaradac:

> As the author told me himself, he owed to chance the great discovery that immortalized his name. We must say at once that these chances would only occur to a man of genius. One day while crossing the court of the Louvre, he noticed children with their ears held to two ends of long pieces of wood, transmitting the noise of small pin strokes on the opposite end. This everyday acoustic experience was a revelation for him. He conceived on the spot the thought of application to heart disease. The next day at his clinic at the Necker hospital, he rolled his appointment notebook, tied it compactly while keeping a central tube, then placed it on a diseased heart. This was the first stethoscope. (my translation of passage quoted by Grmek 1981, p. 113)

Whereas Laennec described himself as using acoustic principles to think of the wooden source analogy, his friend's account described Laennec as serendipitously encountering children listening to a pin scratch wood. The children's game provided a fortuitous source analog that reminded him of his ongoing target problem of effectively listening to patients' chests. In accord with the serendipity model of analogical transfer, the encountered source provided a retrieval cue for the target problem rather than vice versa. The historical record is not adequate to establish which of these accounts is correct, although an authority leans toward Laennec's own story (Grmek 1981). Nevertheless, the two versions of the story are useful for distinguishing between the schema and serendipity models of analogical transfer, and Laennec's discovery under either description qualifies as a technological analogy of great medical importance.

In 1983, Kary Mullis, a biologist at Cetus Corporation in California, invented polymerase chain reaction (PCR), a technology that now has many applications in molecular medicine. PCR is a method in which an enzyme called a polymerase is used to act along a strand of DNA to produce unlimited quantities of selected genetic material for further investigation. The idea for PCR came to him on a drive to his cabin in Mendocino County. He had been looking for a general procedure to identify a single nucleotide at a given position in a DNA molecule. According to Rabinow (1996, p. 96) the discovery came about because Mullis had been experimenting with fractals and other computational procedures that involved iteration and exponential amplification:

> This was the breakthrough moment. His tinkering with fractals and other computer programs had habituated him to the idea of iterative processes. This looping, back and back again, as boring and time consuming as it might be on the level of physical practice, was nearly effortless on the computer. Mullis made the connection between the two realms and saw that the doubling process was a huge advantage because it was exponential.

This discovery appears to fit the standard model of analogical transfer. Wondering about how to solve the target problem of producing large quantities of genetic principle led Mullis to think of a kind of computational problem with which he was familiar. The iterative processes of fractals then provided a source problem that suggested a solution to the target problem. Thus, technological analogies exemplify the standard as well as the schema and serendipity models of analogical transfer.

EDUCATIONAL ANALOGIES

All the analogies I have discussed so far are highly creative ones in which new solutions were suggested for important theoretical, experimental, diagnostic, therapeutic, and technological problems. Much more common, however, are more prosaic educational analogies that function to enable someone who understands something about the nature of disease to convey that information to someone else. Polemics in favor of the bacterial theory of ulcers drew comparisons with other infectious diseases such as smallpox, cystitis, and polio. Zamir (1996) explained why regular exercise is important for healthy hearts by using an extended financial analogy that compares coronary output to bank deposits. Strachan and Read (1996, p. 458) provided an analogy that helps distinguish the roles of different cancer-causing genes: "By analogy with a bus, one can picture the oncogenes as the accelerator and the TS [tumor suppressor] genes as the brake. Jamming the accelerator on (a dominant gain-of-function mutation in an oncogene) or having all the brakes fail (a recessive loss-of-function mutation in a TS gene) will make the bus run out of control." Medical researchers and practitioners can also use analogies to explain new ideas about disease causality to others. Analogies can also be used to give practical advice, as with the following anonymous comparison inspired by mad cow disease. Safe eating is like safe sex: You may be eating whatever it was that what you are eating ate before you ate it.

I have described how analogies are useful in medicine for theoretical, experimental, diagnostic, therapeutic, technological, and educational purposes. The processes of analogical reasoning are not, however, always the same, and different cases of medical analogizing fit different models of analogical transfer, although the standard model in which source analogs are remembered and applied to solve a target problem is probably the most common. The additional examination of historical cases and ongoing medical practice will undoubtedly provide more illustrations of different ways in which analogical transfer can contribute to medical thinking.

SUMMARY

Analogy is a cognitive process that is important in many kinds of creative thinking, so it is not surprising that it also contributes to the growth of medical knowledge. Analogical transfer often fits the standard model in which a source is remembered to solve a target problem. But sometimes it is the target problem that is retrieved, and sometimes the source problem is constructed rather than retrieved. Pasteur, Lister, and other medical researchers have used analogies in their theoretical advances. Analogies have also been useful for designing experiments, suggesting diagnoses, proposing therapeutic treatments, inventing new medical technologies, and enhancing education.

CHAPTER 10

Diseases, Germs, and Conceptual Change

CHAPTERS 7 to 9 on analogy and causal reasoning described cognitive mechanisms by which individual hypotheses can be generated and evaluated. The result of these mechanisms is not only changes in scientists' beliefs but also changes in their concepts. This chapter describes how concepts of disease and their causes have changed over the past one hundred and fifty years. It begins with a review of the nature of concepts and different kinds of conceptual change and then discusses changes in disease concepts. These changes occur primarily in the mental representations of diseases, and germ concepts have undergone similar developments. But germ concepts have also changed with respect to their modes of reference, that is, how they relate to the world. The connections between conceptual changes that are representational (in the mind) and referential (about the world) support the contention of chapter 5 that scientific development is both a physical and a mental process.

CONCEPTUAL CHANGE

What are concepts? In the traditional, purely linguistic view, a concept is given by a definition that specifies necessary and sufficient conditions for its application. According to this view, we should be able to provide definitions, such as X is a disease if and only if ____, and X is tuberculosis if and only if ____. Like other concepts, however, the concept of disease has not succumbed to this kind of linguistic analysis (Reznek 1987). Cognitive science has offered a different view of the nature of concepts, understanding them as mental representations; but the nature of conceptual representations has remained controversial. Theorists have variously proposed that concepts are prototypes, sets of exemplars, or distributed representations in neural networks (for reviews, see Smith 1989; Smith and Medin 1981; Thagard 1992b, chapter 2; Thagard 1996, chapter 4).

Many psychologists have emphasized the role of causal connections in understanding the nature of concepts (Carey 1985; Keil 1989; Medin 1989; Murphy and Medin 1985). The concept of a drunk, for example, is not just a set of prototypical features or typical examples, but it also involves causal relations that can be used to apply the concept in an explanatory fashion: If someone falls into a swimming pool fully clothed, we could say that it happened because he or she is a drunk.

I suggested in chapter 2 that disease concepts have a structure that includes relations among causes, symptoms, and treatments (see Figure 2.1). Understanding a disease concept as a causal structure is consistent with aspects of prototype and exemplar theories of concepts. Patients may have symptoms that approximately match a set of symptoms that typically occur in people with a particular disease. Medical personnel may have in mind particular examples of patients with a particular disease. But a disease concept is not fully captured by a set of typical symptoms or exemplars, because the causal relations are an important part of the conceptual structure.

My account of the structure of disease concepts is consistent with findings by health psychologists that lay theories of illness include elements of symptoms, consequences, temporal course, cause, and cure (see Skelton and Croyle 1991). Michela and Wood (1986) provide a comprehensive review of causal attributions in health and illness. It would be interesting to determine what kinds of conceptual changes must be undertaken by medical students training to be physicians or by laypeople attempting to understand and comply with the treatment of their illnesses

Concepts can change in diverse ways. Thagard (1992b) identifies nine degrees of conceptual change, which are summarized in Table 10.1. Conceptual change is not simply a matter of belief revision, since concepts are not simply collections of beliefs, but they are instead mental structures that are richly organized by means of relations, such as *kind* and *part.* All the major scientific revolutions in the natural sciences—those of Copernicus, Newton, Lavoisier, Darwin, and Einstein, and development of the quantum theory and the theory of plate tectonics—involved major changes in conceptual organization that involved kind and/or part relations (Thagard 1992b). Such changes are far more important, both psychologically and epistemologically, than are mundane changes such as adding new instances or even adding new concepts.

The most radical kind of conceptual change is tree switching, which changes not only the branches of a hierarchy of concepts but also the whole basis on which classifications are made. Such changes are rare, but they occurred in the Darwinian revolution when the theory of evolution by natural selection brought with it a new principle of classification. Before the time of Darwin, species were classified largely in terms of similarity, but the theory of evolution added a more fundamental mode of classification: relatedness in terms of descent. Darwin's trees of organisms were based on a history of descent, not just on similarity. Today, the relatedness of different species can be identified by the degree of similarity of their DNA, providing a genetic, historical basis for classification that often overrules more superficial similarities. The kinds of conceptual change listed in table 10.1 occurred in the

TABLE 10.1

Degrees of Conceptual Change

---

1. Adding a new instance of a concept, for example, a patient who has tuberculosis.
2. Adding a new weak rule, for example, that tuberculosis is common in prisons.
3. Adding a new strong rule that plays a frequent role in problem solving and explanation, for example that people with tuberculosis have *Mycobacterium tuberculosis*.
4. Adding a new part relation, for example, that diseased lungs contain tubercles.
5. Adding a new kind relation, for example, differentiating between pulmonary and miliary tuberculosis.
6. Adding a new concept, for example *tuberculosis* (which replaced the previous terms *phthisis* and *consumption)* or *AIDS*.
7. Collapsing part of a kind hierarchy, and thereby abandoning a previous distinction, for example, realizing that phthisis and scrofula are the same disease: tuberculosis.
8. Reorganizing hierarchies by *branch jumping*, that is, shifting a concept from one branch of a hierarchical tree to another, as in reclassifying tuberculosis as an infectious disease.
9. *Tree switching*, that is, changing the organizing principle of a hierarchical tree, as in classifying diseases in terms of causal agents rather than symptoms.

Source: Adapted from Thagard (1992b, p. 35).

development of the concept of disease, particularly during the transition to the germ theory.

Accounts of conceptual change go back at least as far as the nineteenth-century writings of Georg Hegel and William Whewell but have proliferated since Thomas Kuhn's (1970) work on scientific revolutions. Kuhn (1993, p. 336) now characterizes a scientific revolution in part as "the transition to a new lexical structure, to a revised set of kinds." Terms for these kinds (i.e., *kind terms*) "supply the categories prerequisite to description of and generalization about the world. If two communities differ in their conceptual vocabularies, their members will describe the world differently and make different generalizations about it" (Kuhn 1993, p. 319). The difference is particularly serious if the new set of kind terms overlaps kind terms already in place, since there then can be no straightforward translation between the terms in the two theories (see also Hacking 1993). Buchwald (1992) shows that two competing optical theories in the early nineteenth century worked with taxonomies that cannot be mapped or grafted onto one another.

My discussion of the concepts of disease similarly assumes that scientific categories can be thought of as forming a taxonomic tree, although in medicine the tree is tangled because of the intermingling of physiological and pathogenetic taxonomies (see later). I have described several kinds of changes in the taxonomy of diseases that occurred with the development of the germ theory of disease. It is indeed difficult to translate completely between the humoral and the germ conceptions of disease, because the Hippocratic classification of diseases in terms of bodily locations divides the world up differently from the classification of diseases in terms of microbial causes. Partial translation is nevertheless possible: We can recognize ancient discussions of diseases such as phthisis (tuberculosis) because the symptoms associated with it today are similar to those identified long ago, even if the etiology and taxonomy of the disease have changed dramatically. Like Kuhn (1993, p. 315), who refers to the lexicon as a "mental module," I take conceptual change primarily to be change in mental representations, although I also consider referential change later in this chapter.

CHANGES IN DISEASE CONCEPTS

The authoritative *Cecil Textbook of Medicine* is divided into parts that implicitly classify diseases in two complementary respects: organ systems and pathogenesis. Table 10.2 lists the relevant parts of the textbook. Most of these are organized around physiological systems, such as the cardiovascular and respiratory systems. But there are also parts of the book that group diseases in terms of pathogenetic mechanisms that can affect various organ systems: oncology, metabolic diseases, nutritional diseases, infectious diseases, and so on. Some diseases are naturally discussed in more than one part, as when myocarditis occurs under both cardiovascular diseases and infectious diseases. Modern medical classification thus blends two overlapping taxonomies of disease.

The shift from the humoral to the germ theory of disease described in chapter 2 required a conceptual revolution: The old conceptual and explanatory system was replaced by a radically different one. This revolution is an example of tree switching, in that the whole means of classifying diseases shifted its principle of organization from humors to microbial causes. In contrast, the developments in the twentieth century of concepts of genetic, nutritional, autoimmune, and molecular diseases were more conservative extensions of the nineteenth-century ideas: New causes were introduced without denying that the germ theory was right about the causes of diseases to which it had been successfully applied. There were, however, isolated cases of branch jumping, as when diseases such as beriberi that were suspected of being infectious turned out to be nutritional. Let us now look at changes in the concept of disease more systematically.

The development of the concept of disease illustrates all nine kinds of conceptual change that were distinguished in Table 10.1. I characterize changes as *conservative* if they involve extensions to existing concepts and beliefs, and *nonconservative* if they require a rejection of previous concepts and beliefs. The first kinds of conceptual change—which involve the addition of new instances, such as new cases of tuberculosis and empirical generalizations concerning who tends to get tuberculosis—are usually conservative. Adding a

TABLE 10.2

Organization of *Cecil Textbook of Medicine*

Cardiovascular diseases
Respiratory diseases
Renal diseases
Gastrointestinal diseases
Diseases of the liver, gall bladder, and bile ducts
Hematologic diseases
Oncology
Metabolic diseases
Nutritional diseases
Endocrine and reproductive diseases
Diseases of the bone and bone mineral metabolism
Diseases of the immune system
Musculoskeletal and connective tissue diseases
Infectious diseases
HIV and associated disorders
Diseases caused by protozoa and metazoa
Neurology
Eye diseases
Skin diseases

Source: Wyngaarden et al. (1992).

new causal rule, however, can drastically alter the concept of a disease by changing the links in the causal network for the disease. When Robert Koch showed that tuberculosis is caused by a bacillus, he developed a very different causal network from that of the Hippocratics: Koch's work indicated that the disease is an infection, not an imbalance, that can be treated by killing the microbes that cause the infection, not by overcoming the imbalance. Adding a new causal rule can be conservative if the rule does not clash with a previously held causal rule, but the replacement of the humoral theory by the germ theory required numerous instances of adding nonconservative rules.

Adding a new part relation has usually been a conservative conceptual change in the history of medicine, since finding new parts does not require a rejection of previous views about parts. For example, when Theodor Schwann proposed in 1839 that animals are composed of cells, his new subdivision did not require a rejection of previous views about organs. Identifying new parts, however, can sometimes lead to nonconservative rule addition if the new parts suggest new causal rules, as when the discovery of new organs made novel diagnoses possible.

Adding a new kind relation can be conservative when it involves simply subdividing accepted kinds into finer distinctions, as when diabetes mellitus is divided into two kinds: type I (insulin-dependent) diabetes and type II (non–

insulin dependent, or adult-onset) diabetes. Sometimes, however, adding kind relations involves changing causal rules, as when the germ theory introduced infectious diseases as a new class with causes that differed from those associated with the humoral theory.

Adding a new concept can be conservative when the concept fits with the existing conceptual system. Adding the classes of genetic and nutritional diseases was mostly conservative with respect to the germ theory, since the new concepts applied largely to diseases that had not previously been asserted to be infectious. In contrast, the concept of infectious disease was nonconservative with respect to the humoral theory, since it required rejecting not only previous beliefs but also previous concepts. The modern concepts of blood, phlegm, and bile do not play anything like the explanatory and clinical role that they did for the Hippocratics.

For the germ theory, fever is not itself a disease—as it was for Hippocrates—but only a symptom of infection. Hence, there is no need to include in the taxonomy of diseases a classification of kinds of fever. Abandonment of the fever branch of the disease taxonomy exemplifies the seventh kind of conceptual change listed in Table 10.1, collapsing a kind hierarchy to abandon a previous distinction. This change is clearly nonconservative, requiring the abandonment of previously accepted concepts and beliefs.

Branch jumping—reorganizing hierarchies by shifting a concept from one branch of a hierarchical tree to another branch—is similarly nonconservative. Chapter 3 described how the bacterial theory of ulcers requires reclassification of ulcers as an infectious disease rather than as a disorder due to excess acidity or as a psychosomatic disease due to stress. Similarly, the classification of diseases such as tuberculosis, cholera, rabies, and malaria in terms of their microbial causes shifts these concepts to a new place in the tree of diseases, forcing one to abandon their classification in terms of the kind of fever or superficial symptoms that are produced. Chapter 8 described how many researchers have reclassified spongiform encephalopathies in the new category of prion diseases.

Tree switching, changing the basis on which classifications are made, is nonconservative, since it is linked with the development of new branches that supersede previous classifications. The transition to the germ theory was a case of tree switching, since it introduced classification of diseases in terms of their causes, particularly their microbial causes. Modern medicine no longer classifies diseases in terms of symptoms but rather in terms of their causes and the organ systems affected. Symptoms are related to organ systems, since, for example, a lung disorder has symptoms involving the lungs. But the seat of the disorder and its causes are more fundamental to the classification of diseases than are symptoms. In contrast, dictionaries of symptoms and other books written for laypeople are still organized in terms of symptoms rather than organ systems or causes of disease.

In sum, the transition in the nineteenth century from the humoral theory to the germ theory of disease was highly nonconservative, involving new concepts, new causal rules, and new classifications, as well as the abandonment of old ones. The transition was accomplished largely by the ability of the germ theory to provide a superior new account of the causes and treatments of diseases. In contrast, the twentieth-century expansion of causes of diseases to include genetic, nutritional, autoimmune, and molecular considerations was largely conservative with respect to the germ theory. Some of the diseases that were found to fall under the new classes of disease had previously been suspected of having an infectious origin. For example, when Christiaan Eijkman, a student of Koch, was investigating beriberi, he searched for a microbial cause before serendipitously discovering its connection with polished rice. But I am not aware of any disease confidently classed as infectious that has been shown to have a totally different kind of cause. New causes were introduced without rejecting the established concepts and beliefs about infectious diseases. Harvard Medical School now advocates a "biopsychosocial" model of medicine (Tosteson et al. 1994). The modern trend toward multifactorial theories that envision diseases such as cancers as resulting from complex interactions of genetic, environmental, immunological, and other factors is similarly conservative, except with respect to narrow views that attempt to specify a single cause for each particular disease.

Curiously, the names of some diseases now known to be caused by infectious agents have remained unchanged despite their Hippocratic origins. The bacterial disease cholera was named from the Latin word for the bile humor. The protozoal disease malaria was named from the Italian for bad air. It is not unusual for terms to survive the theories that spawned them: Antoine Lavoisier's term for the part of air that promotes combustion was coined under the erroneous assumption that all acids contain oxygen, and Casimir Funk's 1912 introduction of the term *vitamine* for nutritionally essential organic substances erroneously assumed that these substances all are amines. The term *atom* came from the Greek word for indivisible and survived the discovery of subatomic particles.

All the changes in the concept of disease I have been discussing are changes to mental representations. Carey also takes concepts and beliefs to be mental structures and lists three types of conceptual change (Carey 1992, p. 95). The first, differentiation, occurs when a new distinction is drawn. The development of disease concepts has seen many such differentiations, both in distinguishing between particular diseases, such as measles and smallpox, and in distinguishing between kinds of diseases, such as bacterial infections and viral infections. The second, coalescence, occurs when a distinction is abandoned, as we saw in the abandonment of the Hippocratic distinction between kinds of fever and in the scrapping of the distinction between scrofula and phthisis. In Carey's third kind of conceptual change, simple properties are reanalyzed as relations, as when Newton reanalyzed the concept *weight* as a relation between an object and the earth. Whether there have been medical examples of this kind of conceptual change is unclear.

Chi and her colleagues distinguish between conceptual change within an ontological category and *radical* conceptual change that necessitates a change across ontological categories (Chi 1992; Slotta et al. 1996). She argues that physics education requires radical conceptual change, since students must recategorize familiar concepts such as heat, light, force, and current (which their everyday conceptual systems take to be substances) as events defined by relational constraints between several entities. Radical conceptual change cannot occur merely by adapting or extending a previous conceptual scheme but instead requires constructing a new set of concepts and shifting to it as a whole.

Is change in the concept of disease radical in Chi's sense? Brock (1961, p. 74) suggests that Fracastoro's contagion theory (described in the next section) introduced the concept of an infectious disease as a process rather than as a thing. But the Hippocratics' extensive discussions of the courses and prognoses of diseases suggest that they also considered diseases to fall under the ontological category of process. Chi's fundamental ontological categories are matter (kinds and artifacts), events, and abstractions. For the Hippocratics as well as the nineteenth-century germ theorists, diseases were complex events, not kinds of things or abstractions. The transition to the germ theory of disease therefore did not involve radical conceptual change in Chi's sense. Nevertheless, it did require the sort of replacement mechanism that she describes for radical conceptual change in which a whole new conceptual scheme is constructed, not simply produced by piecemeal modification of the previous humoral scheme. Other interesting discussions of conceptual change include Gentner et al. (1997) and Nersessian (1989, 1992).

REPRESENTATIONAL CHANGES IN GERM CONCEPTS

Accompanying the changes in the concept of disease that were brought about by the germ theory were dramatic changes in concepts that described the infectious agents newly held to be responsible for disease. The development of concepts such as bacteria and viruses involved some of the same kinds of changes so far described for disease concepts.

Although some Hippocratics recognized that consumption (tuberculosis) is contagious, contagion played little role in medical explanations of disease until the work of Girolamo Fracastoro, who was born in Verona about 1478. In 1525, he published a long poem about the newly recognized disease syphilis, and in 1546 he published his major treatise on contagion. Fracastoro did not deny the existence of bodily humors such as phlegm, but he contended that there is a large class of diseases caused by contagion rather than by humoral imbalance. People can contract infections even if their humors are normally balanced. He defined a contagion as a "corruption which develops in the substance of a combination, passes from one thing to another, and is originally caused by infection of the imperceptible particles" (Fracastorius 1930, p. 5). He called the particles the *seminaria* (seeds or seedlets) of contagion. (I translate Fracastoro's "seminaria" as "seeds" rather than the customary but anachronistic "germs.") He described how contagion can occur by direct contact, by indirect contact via clothes and other substances, and by long-distance transmission. He also stated that diseases can arise within an individual spontaneously. The differences between diseases are explained by their having different "active principles," (i.e., different seeds). Fracastoro distinguished between different kinds of fevers in part on the basis of their being caused by different kinds of contagion. Rather than abandoning the humoral theory, he blended this theory with his contagion theory, suggesting that seeds for different diseases have different analogies (affinities) for different humors. The principles of syphilis, for example, have an affinity with thick phlegm, whereas those of elephantiasis have an affinity with black bile.

Just as Fracastoro's contagion theory of disease postulates different causes than the humoral theory, it also recommends different treatments. Cure comes not from restoring a bodily imbalance but from destroying or expelling the seeds of contagion. Remedies that destroy the seeds of contagion include extreme heat and cold, whereas evacuation of the seeds can be brought about by bowel movements, urination, sweating, blood letting, and other methods. Methods of treatment thus overlap with those advocated by the Hippocratics, although Fracastoro urged that blood letting not be used for contagious diseases that arise from without, as opposed to those that are spontaneously generated from within. The *seminaria* produce an infection that can be treated by destroying or expelling them.

According to Nutton (1990), Fracastoro's theory of contagion was respectfully received by his contemporaries, although they tended to assimilate his views to the Galenist metaphor of "seeds of disease," which did not, unlike Fracastoro's view, assume that such seeds are infectious agents transmitted from one person to another. Because no one had observed the *seminaria* postulated by Fracastoro, his hypothesis had no obvious advantage over Hippocratic assumptions that noxious airs (miasmas) rather than germs are a main source of epidemic diseases. The dominant view continued to be that diseases arise because of humor-altering miasmas. Fracastoro had little influence after 1650, although interest in his work revived in the nineteenth century with the emergence of the modern germ theory.

Microscopic living creatures were first observed in 1674 by Antony van Leeuwenhoek. Examining a sample of lake water with a simple microscope, he observed "very many little animalcules"; his descriptions apply to what are now called protozoa (Dobell 1958, p. 110). In 1676, Leeuwenhoek observed many animalcules in water in which pepper had been standing for some weeks, including some "incredibly small" animalcules that were evidently bacteria.

Although we can say that Leeuwenhoek discovered protozoa and bacteria, these concepts did not originate with him, for he wrote only of animalcules that differed in their sizes and parts. Leeuwenhoek never associated the animalcules he observed with the causation of disease. The concept of germ that arose in the nineteenth century was both biological and medical: A germ is a biological organism that can cause disease. The Fracastoro concept of *seminaria* was medical but not biological; Leeuwenhoek's concept of *animalcule* was biological but not medical. Fracastoro and Leeuwenhoek both introduced new concepts that retrospectively can be seen as ancestors of modern microbiology but were very different from their related current concepts.

In the twelfth edition (1767) of the *Systema Naturae*, Carolus Linnaeus assigned all the animalcules then known to three genera, *Volvo, Furia*, and *Chaos* (Linné 1956). The entities that Leeuwenhoek had observed were termed *infusoria* in the eighteenth century because they were observed in infusions (solutions) of decaying organic matter. Linnaeus lumped all the infusoria to a single species, *Chaos infusorium* (Bulloch 1979, p. 37). The term *bacterium* was introduced by Gottfried in 1829.

Modern microbiology began with the French chemist Louis Pasteur, who in 1857 discovered that lactic acid fermentation is caused by a microorganism, yeast. Previously, fermentation was believed to be the result of decomposition of a substance, not the effect of an organism such as yeast. In 1861, Pasteur announced that the ferment that produces butyric acid is an infusorium ("infusoire," Brock 1961, p. 265). The anaerobic bacteria observed by Pasteur were small cylindrical rods about .002 millimeter in diameter. This discovery, as well as subsequent work by Pasteur, Koch, and others on the involvement of microorganisms in disease, led to an explosion of work that resulted, by the end of the nineteenth century, in the identification of many different kinds of bacteria and protozoa. It also led to demonstrations that many important diseases such as tuberculosis and malaria are caused by microbes. (The term "microbe" was introduced in 1878 by Sédillot.)

Attempts were made to identify microbes that were responsible for diseases such as rabies and smallpox, but the agents in these cases were what we now call viruses, which are too small to be seen through an optical microscope. The term *virus* originally meant "poison," and any cause of disease, including Fracastorios's *seminaria*, could be referred to as a virus. In 1884, Charles Chamberland used filtration through a porous vase of porcelain to purify water of microbes, but in 1892 Dmitri Ivanovski was surprised to find that a filtered extract from diseased tobacco plants could cause disease in previously healthy plants. In 1898, Löffler and Frosch conjectured that hoof and mouth disease is caused by "a previously undiscovered agent of disease, so small as to pass through the pores of a filter retaining the smallest known bacteria"

(Lechevalier and Solotorovsky 1974, pp. 284–285). The conjectured poison became known as a "filterable virus." After 1915, when Frederick Twort showed that bacteria can be attacked by filterable viruses, the concept of a virus as an ultramicroscopic organism became established. In 1935, Wendell Stanley presented crystallographic evidence that tobacco mosaic virus is a protein. During the 1930s, the electron microscope was developed, and in 1939 Kausch, Pfankuch, and Ruska used it to describe the appearance of the tobacco mosaic virus. Thus, the use of the term *virus* evolved gradually from one concerning any disease-causing poison to one concerning very small microorganisms detected by electron microscopes.

When Leeuwenhoek introduced the term *animalcule*, he added to his mental apparatus a new concept that differentiated the newly observed entities from larger animals. Concepts need not be formed directly by observation, however, but can be formed as part of the generation of explanatory hypotheses. Fracastoro's concept of *seminaria* did not refer to any entity he had observed but rather to one he had postulated to explain contagion. Similarly, the concept of a filterable virus initially concerned a hypothetical entity, although viruses later were identified by electron microscopy.

After Pasteur, Joseph Lister, and others showed the medical significance of bacteria in the 1860s, great progress was made in identifying new kinds of bacteria and in demonstrating their roles in a host of diseases, including diphtheria, tuberculosis, and cholera. By the end of the 1870s, people no longer spoke of *the* bacteria but of different bacteria (Bulloch 1979, p. 203). In place of the general concepts of animalcule and infusorium, concepts referring to particular kinds of bacteria and protozoa were developed, and the concept of microbe was introduced to reunify the plethora of newly differentiated concepts. The taxonomy of bacteria was important for the development of the germ theory of disease: If one bacterium could unpredictably turn into another kind, then it would be difficult to accept the fact that a specific disease was caused by a specific bacterium (Brock 1988, p. 73). Today, more than two thousand species of bacteria have been identified, along with many species of protozoa.

The proliferation of microbiological concepts did not simply involve extension of existing classification but often required revision of kind relations. Leeuwenhoek and the eighteenth-century taxonomists classified bacteria and other infusoria as animals. In 1852, however, Perty contended that some of the infusoria are *animal-plants*, and Ferdinand Cohn argued in 1854 that bacteria of the genus *Vibriona* are plants analogous to algae. In 1857, the German botanist Karl Nageli proposed that bacteria should be regarded as a class of their own within the vegetable kingdom, for which he coined the term Schizomycetes, or "fission fungi" (Collard 1976, p. 151). Today, in the widely used five kingdom classification, bacteria are no longer classed with fungi, but rather with the cyanobacteria (blue-green algae) in the kingdom Monera.

Reclassification of viruses has been even more complex. Originally, *virus* meant "slime" or "poison," but only at the end of the nineteenth century did it start to acquire the meaning of "infectious agent." By the 1940s, the electron microscope made it possible to discern the structure of many kinds of viruses, which are particles consisting only of DNA or RNA (but not both) and a protein shell. Unlike bacteria, which are living cells, viruses cannot reproduce on their own but rather only when they are parasites in living cells. When Pasteur and other early researchers attempted to identify the cause of diseases such as rabies and smallpox, they thought they were looking for a kind of bacteria, but viruses turned out to be a much smaller and simpler kind of entity. Hundreds of kinds of viruses have been identified. By 1950, viruses were soundly differentiated from bacteria, and the field of virology split off from bacteriology. The mental representations of microbiologists reflect these differences, and hundreds of kinds of viruses are now distinguished based on their structure as revealed by electron microscopy. Viruses "cannot logically be placed in either a strictly biochemical or in a strictly biological category; they are too complex to be macromolecules in the ordinary sense and too divergent in their physiology and manner of replication be conventional living organisms" (Hughes 1977, p. 106). Virologists are wont to say: Viruses are viruses.

The reclassification of bacteria first as Schizomycetes and then Monera, and the reclassification of viruses as a unique kind of entity are examples of branch jumping, the movement of a concept from one branch of a taxonomic tree to another. The development of concepts of bacteria and viruses does not seem to have involved a radical change in classificatory practices, although after 1908 pathogenicity was admitted as a taxonomic criterion for bacteria (Collard 1976, p. 153). The empirical classification is designed to aid the differentiation between medically and industrially important species and others. Chapter 3 described branch jumping in the development of the concept of *Helicobacter pylori*, and chapter 8 described the shift from classifying the causes of kuru and scrapie as slow viruses to classifying them as prions.

In sum, conceptual change in microbiology has involved the formation of many new mental representations that correspond to terms such as *animalcule*, *bacteria*, and *virus*. Concept formation often involved differentiation, as new kinds of entity were distinguished from ones previously known. In addition, the organization of microbiological concepts has changed dramatically over time, as new kinds of infectious agents have been identified and existing kinds have been reclassified in terms of higher order kinds. The concept of infection has also changed, as the modern meaning of invasion by microorganisms has replaced the older, vaguer meaning of infection as staining or pollution. Today, infectious diseases can be differentiated as bacterial infections or viral infections, just as "germs" can be differentiated as bacteria or viruses. Thus, mental representations of germ concepts and the concept of infection changed in tandem with changes in the concept of disease.

GERMS: REFERENTIAL CHANGE

The meaning of a concept is not just a matter of its relation to other concepts but also of its relation to the world. Kitcher (1993) describes conceptual change, not in terms of mental representations but in terms of *modes of reference*, which are causal connections between a term and an object that make it the case that the term refers to the object. He describes three types of mode of reference: *descriptive*, when the speaker uses a description to pick out an object to which a term is intended to refer; *baptismal*, when a speaker ostensively applies a term to a particular present object; and *conformist*, when a speaker's usage is parasitic on the usage of others who have established the reference of a term either descriptively or baptismally. A term may have multiple modes of reference, which together comprise its *reference potential.* According to Kitcher (1993, p. 103), conceptual change is change in reference potential.

The germ theory undoubtedly brought with it new modes of reference for disease terms. Tuberculosis could now be described as the disease caused by the tubercle bacillus. Disease concepts did not change completely, however, since the descriptive modes of reference associated with familiar observable symptoms did not change. Terms for the various microbes that cause disease had baptismal modes of reference that occurred when researchers such as Koch first observed them under the microscope.

When Fracastoro described *seminaria* as the causes of contagion, he used a verbal description that was intended to refer to agents of disease. Microbiologists from Leeuwenhoek on, however, were able to fix the reference of terms for microorganisms baptismally by pointing to examples of the new kinds of microorganisms that were being discovered. Their ability to do this depended on the development of a series of technological advances that now illustrate the crucial role of instruments in conceptual change in microbiology.

Why was Leeuwenhoek the first to discover the tiny "animalcules" that we now call bacteria? Others in his time were using microscopes to look at previously unobserved phenomena, but Leeuwenhoek developed his own techniques of microscope construction that were unrivaled for decades afterward. He was able to see numerous sorts of previously unidentified organisms. Here is Leeuwenhoek's own description of the first observation of bacteria, which took place in 1676 as the accidental result of an attempt to discover why pepper is hot to the tongue:

> I did now place anew about ⅓ ounce of whole pepper in water, and set it in my
> closet, with no other design than to soften the pepper, that I could better study
> it. . . . This pepper having lain about three weeks in the water, . . . I saw therein,
> with great wonder, incredibly many very little animalcules, of divers sorts. . . .

The fourth sort of little animals, which drifted among the three sorts aforesaid, were incredibly small; nay, so small, in my sight, that I judged that even if 100 of these very wee animals lay stretched out one against another, they could not reach to the length of a grain of course sand. (excerpts from Dobell 1958, pp. 132–133)

Observation of bacteria through a microscope is not easy, both because of the difficulty of producing accurate lenses and because of the need to focus on the specimens where bacteria exist. Microscopes that reduced aberration sufficiently to facilitate observation of bacteria were not available until the 1820s. Fixing the referent of concepts that referred to different kinds of bacteria depended on these advances in microscopy.

Other experimental techniques were also required for the development of bacteriology (Collard 1976). Through the 1870s, it was difficult to obtain pure cultures that contained only one kind of bacterium, since liquid solutions tended to contain many kinds of bacteria. But in 1881, Koch developed a technique of growing bacteria on cut potatoes, and the next year agar was introduced as a solid medium for culturing bacteria. The identification of many medically important bacteria in the next few years used these new techniques, as did the culturing of *H. pylori* described in chapter 3.

The transparency of bacteria makes them difficult to observe, but staining techniques have provided powerful ways of determining their presence and structure. Vegetable stains were applied first to bacteria in 1869, and improved techniques, including Gram's technique of counter staining, were developed over the next decades. Like culturing in solid media, staining is an important aid in fixing the reference of terms for new kinds of bacteria. Culturing and staining enabled Koch to discover the bacterium responsible for tuberculosis:

On the basis of my extensive observations, I consider it as proved that in all tuberculous conditions of man and animals there exists a characteristic bacterium which I have designated as the tubercle bacillus, which has specific properties which allow it to be distinguished from all other microorganisms. (Koch, quoted in Brock 1988, p. 121)

The baptismal mode of reference to the tubercle bacillus thus depended on the development of new experimental techniques.

New techniques were also crucial for the referential development of concepts concerning viruses. Filtration techniques in the 1880s made possible the differentiation of viruses from bacteria, which were too large to pass through the filters. At this point, the only mode of reference for filterable viruses was descriptive: Virus was whatever passed through the filters and caused disease. After 1920, centrifuges were increasingly used to isolate viruses and to estimate their sizes based on centrifugation times and the force of gravity. A few very large viruses can be identified with optical microscopes, but the baptismal fixing of reference of most concepts of viruses requires use of the electron microscope, which also allowed researchers to determine the structure of bacteria. Before 1939, when Kausche, Pfankuch, and Ruska first used the electron microscope for visualization of a virus, the mode of reference was descriptive, as in "the virus of measles." The third type of mode of reference defined by Kitcher (1993) is conformist, based on the usage of others who have established the reference of a term either descriptively or baptismally. For most people, the reference of concepts such as *bacteria* and *virus* is fixed in this way, since they have neither seen such entities themselves nor been given an accurate description.

REPRESENTATION, REFERENCE, AND CONCEPTUAL CHANGE

How are Kitcher's three modes of reference—descriptive, baptismal, and conformist—related to representational changes that involve concept formation, differentiation, and reclassification (branch jumping)? Descriptive modes of reference that involve words and verbal descriptions are easily cast in terms of mental representation by supposing that thinkers have (1) mental concepts that correspond to words and (2) proposition-like representations that correspond to descriptions. People presumably have a mental representation for the concept *bacteria* that makes possible their use of the word *bacteria*. With respect to description, the mental representation view of conceptual change is currently richer than the referential view, since it pays attention to the kind relations of concepts. But ideas such as differentiation and reclassification could be reframed in terms of a verbal lexicon rather than a mental lexicon by taking *kind* as a relation among verbal terms rather than as mental structures. Given the theoretical richness of taking concepts as mental representations, there is no reason to prefer the discussion of terms as words rather than as concepts.

But the reference potential view of conceptual change does have an advantage over the mental representation in its ability to facilitate an understanding of the relation between representations and the world. The baptismal mode of reference operated repeatedly in the history of microbiology—from Leeuwenhoek fixing the reference of *animalcule* to Koch fixing the reference of *tubercle bacillus* to electron microscopists fixing the reference of *tobacco mosaic virus*. This mode of reference is best viewed not as a single act but as a matter of ongoing interaction with the world using instruments and experimental techniques. Koch not only baptized the tubercle bacillus, but he also photographed and showed how to culture it and transmit it to laboratory animals. This contribution was more than description, and more than baptism: It was development of replicable physical procedures for interacting with the entity referred to by the term (or concept) *tubercle bacillus*. Changes in such procedures and attendant new baptismal episodes are aspects of conceptual change that are not captured by concentration solely on mental representation.

When concepts are formed purely descriptively, for example, when seminaria are characterized as the seeds of disease, conceptual change can be viewed in terms of mental structures. But when concepts are formed ostensively as the result of interactions with the world, we have to understand conceptual change in terms of reference as well as representation. Differentiation is not only conceptual: Entities can be differentiated into different classes if observation makes them sufficiently distinguishable that they can be dubbed independently. Chapter 5 described the important role of the electron microscope in displaying Warren's gastric bacteria in sufficient detail that they could be differentiated from *Campylobacter* bacteria.

Although changes in baptismal reference fixation are important to understanding the development of germ concepts, they are not so directly relevant to understanding the development of disease concepts. Because diseases involve complexes of symptoms, there is no entity that one can identify ostensively. Reference to diseases is fixed descriptively in terms of their symptoms or causes, although reference to symptoms and microbial causes can be fixed baptismally. The mental representation approach has also tended to neglect the social nature of conceptual change that is implicit in Kitcher's conformist mode of reference. Even from the perspective of mental representation, conceptual change is a social as well as psychological phenomenon.

Although representational accounts of conceptual change do not tell the whole story, there remains ample reason to describe conceptual change in part as change in mental representations, especially kind relations. Conceptual change is clearly both representational and referential, since the meaning of concepts is a function of both how they relate to each other and how they relate to the world. A full theory of conceptual change must integrate its representational, referential, and social aspects. The next three chapters consider the social processes that are involved in the growth of scientific knowledge.

SUMMARY

Conceptual change comes in varying degrees, from the addition of new concepts to the revision of existing concepts to the revolutionary replacement of a whole set of concepts. Particularly in the transition from the humoral theory of disease to the germ theory, medicine has undergone important kinds of conceptual change, including the reclassification of diseases and infectious agents. Conceptual change is change in mental representations, but it is also change in how terms are used to refer to things in the world. For germ concepts, representational change was intimately linked to referential change, through the use of microscopes to observe new infectious agents.

Part Four

SOCIAL PROCESSES

CHAPTER 11

Collaborative Knowledge

As CHAPTER 6 described, the social process of collaboration among research-ers was essential to the development of the bacterial theory of ulcers. This chapter assesses more generally how collaboration contributes to the develop-ment of scientific knowledge. My concern with collaboration is both descrip-tive—how it is part of science—and prescriptive—why it is part of how sci-ence should be. I want simultaneously to describe why scientists collaborate and to evaluate the epistemic contribution of collaboration, that is, how it en-hances the development of knowledge. This chapter distinguishes four differ-ent kinds of collaboration, which can be assessed using Goldman's five stan-dards for appraising epistemic practices. A sixth standard is proposed to help understand the importance of theoretical collaborations in cognitive science and other fields. The aim of this chapter is to answer such questions as these: How prevalent is collaborative knowledge? Why do scientists collaborate? What kinds of collaboration are most productive? Why is collaboration in the humanities much rarer than in the sciences?

THE PREVALENCE OF COLLABORATION

In April 1994, a group of 450 physicists centered at Fermilab presented evi-dence for the existence of the top quark, an important theoretical construct of the standard model of particles and forces. Although the size of this group is unusual, the collaborative nature of their work is not. In the natural and social sciences, it has become much more the norm than the exception to have work produced by two or more cooperating scientists. Figure 11.1 graphs the per-centages of multiauthored papers in the physical and biological sciences, the social sciences, and the humanities up to the 1950s. By that time, eighty-three percent of papers in selected journals in the physical and biological sciences were collaborative efforts. In the social sciences, the number was thirty-two percent, whereas in the humanities the number remained relatively constant at one or two percent. The trend has continued in recent decades: Figure 11.2 shows the percentages of multiauthored papers for selected journals in differ-ent fields for 1992. In *Physical Review Letters*, eighty-eight percent of papers were multiauthored, and in *Cognitive Psychology* seventy-five percent of pa-pers involved collaboration.

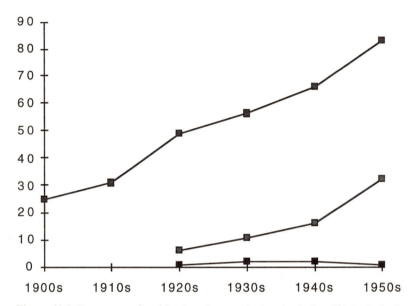

Figure 11.1. Percentage of multiauthored papers in the physical and biological sciences (top line), social sciences (middle line), and humanities (bottom line) from the 1900s to the 1950s. Based on data from Merton (1973), p. 547.

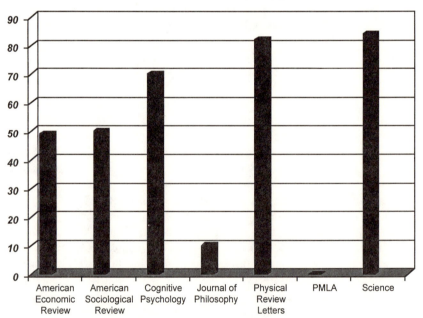

Figure 11.2. Percentage of multiauthored papers in selected journals in 1992. PMLA is the *Proceedings of the Modern Language Association*, whose 1992 volume had no collaborative papers.

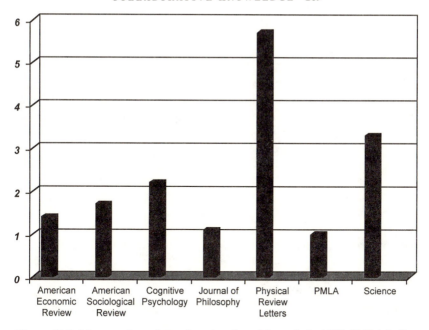

Figure 11.3. Mean number of coauthors in selected journals in 1992. PMLA is *Proceedings of the Modern Language Association.*

Research in the sciences is much more collaborative than work in the humanities. Although philosophers gain greatly from talking with each other, philosophical writings are rarely collaborative. In the 1992 volume of the *Journal of Philosophy*, for example, only three of twenty-seven papers have two authors, and only one has three authors; the rest are single authored. The 1993 volume of the same journal has only one collaborative article. In contrast, of the sixteen papers in the 1992 volume of *Cognitive Psychology*, only four are single authored, whereas six have two authors and the rest have from three to six authors. Similarly, of the 161 papers published in the proceedings of the 1994 Conference of the Cognitive Science Society, only fifty-two are single authored, whereas seventy-one have two authors and thirty-eight have between three and eight authors. Even more extreme, in the January to April 1992 volume of *Physical Review Letters*, only sixty-seven of 558 contributions are single authored, around 12%. One hundred and sixty-eight papers have two authors, and 254 have from three to five authors. Six papers have more than one hundred authors, with the largest total being 291. Figure 11.3 shows the mean number of coauthors in journals in different fields. By looking more closely at different kinds of collaboration, we can start to explain why combined work is so common in the sciences but rare in the humanities.

THE NATURE OF COLLABORATION

Not all collaborations are alike. There are at least four different kinds of collaboration, which reflect the different backgrounds and roles of the collaborators:

1. Employer-Employee. This is the weakest form of collaboration, in which an employer simply tells an employee to perform a task that the employer knows how to do but does not want to spend the time on. Examples of such tasks include running experiments, writing computer programs, constructing apparatuses, and so on. Technicians and research assistants do not normally make sufficient contribution to be considered coauthors, but a talented assistant may become an apprentice as described in the next category.

2. Teacher-Apprentice. This kind of collaboration is similar to the previous one in that there is an asymmetry of knowledge and status, but it has a different goal. Apprentices do not merely perform work that the instructing researchers lack time for, but the apprentices also aim to acquire the skills that will enable them to do the work themselves. Experimental psychologists, for example, typically work closely with graduate students who help design and run experiments. Designing experiments and statistically interpreting the results are complex skills that are not typically learned by reading books or taking classes but rather by working on projects with experienced researchers.

3. Peer—similar. Sometimes researchers of similar knowledge, interests, and status find it advantageous to work together. Perhaps the most famous collaboration of this century is the work by Francis Crick and James Watson on the structure of DNA. In psychology, there have been such productive duos as Allan Newell and Herbert Simons and Daniel Kahneman and Amos Tversky. Of course, *similar* does not mean *identical*: Any two researchers even in the same field have somewhat different knowledge and skills to bring to a collaboration. But we can place in this category collaborations that involve people whose training has been substantially alike.

4. Peer—different. Cross-disciplinary research is more likely to bring together researchers with similar goals but different knowledge and skills. In cognitive science, for example, a typical collaboration involves a psychologist and a computer scientist (see other examples later). The former has expertise in theoretical and experimental psychology, including knowledge of how to do experiments, whereas the latter has computational expertise including knowledge of how to build programs that simulate aspects of thinking. Collaborations within physics may involve combinations of theoretical and experimental physicists who have very different kinds of skills.

Of course, the boundaries between these four kinds of collaboration can blur. A clever employee can turn into an apprentice, and a successful teacher-apprentice relationship should gradually become closer to a peer-similar collaboration. Researchers from disparate fields may start out as peer-different collaborators but become more similar as each learns more about the other's field. But these four different kinds of collaboration provide a start at addressing the question of what makes collaboration worthwhile.

GOLDMAN'S STANDARDS FOR EPISTEMIC APPRAISAL

The prevalence of collaboration strongly suggests that scientists must have good epistemic reasons for working together, but what are these? In the novel *Cantor's Dilemma*, written by a Stanford University chemist, a research scientist begins to suspect that his star postdoctoral fellow has been fabricating data on an important experiment (Djerassi 1989). This story illustrates one of the perils of collaboration, which can increase error as well as productivity. In considering the merits of different kinds of collaboration, we need to assess the occurrence of losses as well as gains.

Alvin Goldman has developed a set of standards for assessing epistemic practices. He advocates *veritism* as the principal approach to social epistemology, taking the goal of truth as central to all intellectual pursuits. All his standards of appraisal for evaluating a social practice are concerned with truth (Goldman 1992, p. 195):

1. The *reliability* of a practice is measured by the ratio of truths to total number of beliefs fostered by the practice.

2. The *power* of a practice is measured by its ability to help cognizers find true answers to the questions that interest them.

3. The *fecundity* of a practice is its ability to lead to large numbers of true beliefs for *many* practitioners.

4. The *speed* of a practice is how quickly it leads to true answers.

5. The *efficiency* of a practice is how well it limits the cost of getting true answers.

Before proceeding to apply these five standards to the four kinds of collaboration listed in the previous section, it is useful to reframe the standards in less veritistic terms. Many scientists would blanch at having their findings described as "truths," since the truth of scientific claims gets sorted out only in the long run, as experiments and theories accumulate. Hence, if our goal is to understand why scientists collaborate, we need to describe what they do according to more short-term goals than truth. As an alternative vocabulary, let us describe scientists as seeking *results*, which can include both empirical results consisting of experimental or observational findings as well as theoretical results that consist of the development of theories that explain the empirical results. The criteria for considering something as a result are less stringent and metaphysical than those for counting something as a truth; as a first approximation, we can consider an empirical or theoretical claim a result if it is acceptable by a scientist's peers. Unanimous acceptance by one's peers is not required; perhaps a minimal requirement is that it should be publishable in a good, peer-reviewed journal. Ultimately, we want the results to be true, but in understanding everyday scientific practice we do not want to have to wait the years or decades that might be required for full validation.

The opposite of a result is an *error*, an experimental or theoretical claim that would tend to be rejected by well-informed peers. We can now reframe Goldman's standards as follows:

1. The *reliability* of a practice is measured by the ratio of results to total number of results and errors fostered by the practice.

2. The *power* of a practice is measured by its ability to help cognizers find results that answer the questions that interest them.

3. The *fecundity* of a practice is its ability to lead to large numbers of results for *many* practitioners.

4. The *speed* of a practice is how quickly it leads to results.

5. The *efficiency* of a practice is how well it limits the cost of getting results.

The connection between these standards and Goldman's original veritistic ones is that what I call results are what scientists generally take to be true, and what I call errors are what scientists generally take to be false. From the perspective of scientific realism (e.g., chapter 5 of this book; Thagard 1988 [chapter 8]), results often *are* true, and errors often *are* false. I agree with Goldman that science seeks and sometimes achieves truth, so the title of this chapter is legitimately Collaborative Knowledge rather than just Collaborative Belief. But for understanding the epistemic value of collaboration, we need shorter term, more readily assessable standards than veritistic ones.

The question now becomes this: How do the different kinds of collaboration affect the reliability, power, fecundity, speed, and efficiency of scientific research?

WHY COLLABORATE? GAINS AND (OCCASIONAL) LOSSES

Employer-Employee

When a scientific researcher hires an employee such as a laboratory technician, research assistant, or computer programmer, it is probably unreasonable to expect increased reliability. Unless the employee has esoteric skills and tasks, most of what he or she does could probably be done at least as well by the

researcher. Reliability, therefore, is not the most relevant standard for appreciating this kind of collaboration. The researcher presumably cares enough about
reliability to not want an employee whose work is dramatically increasing the
error rate; however, accepting a somewhat higher error rate will normally have
to be an acceptable tradeoff for not doing everything by oneself. It is possible,
however, that some tasks will actually be done more reliably by an employee
than by the researcher, who may, for example, not be as good a computer
programmer as a young assistant.

With good employees, potential losses in reliability are more than compensated for by gains in power, speed, and efficiency. Division of labor in which
employees such as technicians do simpler or more time-consuming tasks allows researchers more time to work on experimental or theoretical projects.
The effect should then be that of the researcher obtaining more desired results
(power), and obtaining them faster (speed). Hiring an employee does increase
the cost of research, thereby potentially reducing efficiency, but not nearly as
much as hiring an additional researcher. Improvements in power and speed are
not a sure result of hiring an employee, since the researcher has to spend time
training and supervising the employee. Initially, the time spent may exceed the
time that a researcher might have required to do a task alone, but in the long
run the time and effort required to monitor the employee should drop well
below the amount of researcher time and effort expended. Fecundity—the
question of getting many results for many people—does not seem to be relevant to assessing employer-employee collaborations.

Teacher-Apprentice

In many of the natural and social sciences, graduate students are an essential
part of the conduct of research. In the humanities, graduate students typically
pursue projects unconnected to the research of their advisor, who accordingly
treat them at best with benign neglect. In contrast, in fields such as experimental physics and psychology, graduate students are often a crucial part of the
research team, with primary responsibility for the collection of empirical results. Students may work with advisors on experimental design and put in long
hours collecting data. As with employees, researchers find it worthwhile to
collaborate with graduate students, because the gains in power and speed may
compensate for possible losses in reliability and efficiency. Reliability can
suffer, because newly trained students may not know as much as established
researchers about how to avoid mistakes, and the cost of research is increased
by the need to fund the students. But effective graduate students, who assume
time-consuming tasks that would otherwise have to be done by a researcher,
can greatly contribute to more and faster results. This contribution involves

power (how much gets done) as well as speed (how fast it gets done). Having an apprentice perform such labor-intensive tasks as running experiments and writing computer programs can enable researchers to complete tasks that they would never have attempted otherwise.

Teacher-apprentice collaborations differ from employer-employee collaborations in a crucial respect. Researchers work with graduate students not only to increase their own productivity but also to *train* the students. Training in experimental work is much more complicated than imparting knowledge of the sort that is available in print. Effective experiments and their statistical analysis usually involve a wealth of techniques that can be acquired only by working with someone who already has such experience. Conducting science requires much more than knowledge that something is true; it requires knowledge *how* to design experiments, construct apparatuses, and interpret complex data statistically. The goal of apprenticeship is not simply to enhance an advisor's career but to bring students to the point where they can carry out effective research on their own. In Goldman's terms, teacher-apprentice collaborations have the potential to increase fecundity, since they produce new researchers who can go on to obtain results of their own.

Teacher-apprentice collaborations are the most common type in the sciences, but they are rare in the humanities. One reason for this discrepancy is that researchers in the sciences often have grant money that they can use to hire graduate students as research assistants. Humanities graduate students are in contrast typically funded (if at all) by teaching assistantships that do not involve working closely with a supervisor. A second reason is that the humanities do not obviously lend themselves to the kind of division of labor that is natural in sciences, in which students can be assigned time-consuming tasks in data collection. Unlike work in the humanities, many projects in the natural and social sciences are decomposable in ways that make it possible to apportion different parts of them to different people. A third reason why collaboration is rare in the humanities is simply tradition: Young assistant professors never worked collaboratively with their advisors, so they do not expect to work collaboratively with their students. Effective collaboration requires communication and organizational skills to establish a useful division of labor and maintain progress. In the sciences, in which collaboration is entrenched, these skills can be learned implicitly as a part of graduate training, in which an effective advisor provides a role model for how students can conduct collaborative research when they have their own students.

The best apprenticeships turn into full-fledged collaborations, as students develop into equals with their advisors. In physics, it is not unusual for students to continue to work with their advisors after graduation as a member of the large research teams that are increasingly found in that field. In contrast, psychologists need to cut loose from their students, since the students will otherwise not establish a strong enough research record on their own to obtain tenure and grants. Young psychologists, unlike young physicists, are expected to establish their own track record, whereas in physics the costs of research are often so great that independence would be too much to expect of a recent PhD graduate.

The issue of how independent students eventually need to become from their advisors exemplifies a difficult ethical issue in collaborations: the apportionment of credit and blame. Obviously, of the 450 names on a physics paper, not all researchers made equal contribution to the work described. Some may have made no intellectual contribution at all but are included simply because they are a part of the team or managed the enterprise. It becomes difficult to know who to reward for desired results, or who to blame for the production of error. Notoriously, credit for work done jointly by students and advisors goes unduly to the established researchers. Merton terms this the *Matthew effect*, from the Gospel according to St. Matthew: "For unto every one that hath will be given, and he shall have abundance: but from he that hath not shall be taken away even that which he hath" (Merton 1973, p. 445). Many psychology departments require that candidates for tenure develop a research program independent of that of their PhD supervisor. Although this requirement can be helpful in permitting an assessment of a researcher's independent capabilities, it sometimes leads to premature termination of fruitful collaborations. The assumption is that young researchers cannot earn the sort of credit they need for promotion if they are working with their original supervisors. This assumption is clearly too strong, since there are collaborations between students and advisors in which it is clear that the student made most of the contribution. Problems of apportionment of credit also arise with collaborations among equals.

My discussion has been largely from the perspective of established researchers. Graduate students and junior researchers may have different and less pleasant reasons for engaging in collaborations, for example, to secure funding and research resources. Collaborations of the employer-employee and teacher-apprentice types sometimes involves power issues that differ from the epistemic ones discussed in this paper.

Peer—Similar

Whereas employer-employee and teacher-apprentice collaborations involve people with substantial differences in knowledge and status, a less common kind of collaboration brings together established researchers with similar knowledge and interests. What would two researchers gain by working together rather than independently? It might be expected that the time spent in coordination and communication would merely subtract from time that could be spent on individual projects. In the branch of computer science concerned with parallel computation, n processors working together in a network are expected to produce less than an n-times increase in efficiency. Improvement is expected to be sublinear because of the efforts required for communication and coordination. If researchers have similar backgrounds, what can they gain by working with each other?

Surprisingly, computer simulations have shown that the sublinear expectation does not hold for groups of complex agents who work on tasks that require some degree of intelligence (Clearwater, et al. 1991). The task used in the simulations in this study was cryptarithmetic, which requires decoding letters into numbers in a way that makes true mathematical equations, such as WOW + HOT = TEA. For example, the sum DONALD + GERALD = ROBERT has a solution given by A=4, B=3, D=5, E=9, G=1, L=8, N=6, O=2, R=7, and T=0. Clearwater et al. developed a computer system that has one hundred agents working on such tasks cooperatively. Cooperation takes place by having each agent who is randomly generating and testing solutions announce any progress he or she is making to the other agents by communicating a "hint" to the other agents. The interesting result was that n agents communicating in this way could together solve cryptarithmetic problems more than n times faster than all the agents working alone. The cause of the superlinear improvement seems to be that hints effectively reduce the size of the search space: Having agents start off at different locations increases the likelihood that some will find hints that are worth communicating to other agents and that will reduce their subsequent search. Two heads working together can thus be more than twice as good as two heads working alone. Goldman's standards provide a way of seeing how something similar can hold in scientific research.

First, consider reliability. Because it is easier to identify blunders in others than in oneself, peer-similar collaborations can improve reliability by virtue of team members noticing mistakes that they would otherwise miss. Reliability can occasionally suffer, however, if it leads to increased sloppiness based in overconfidence in one's collaborators. Work on decision making has identified the phenomenon of *groupthink*: that members of a group can sometimes end up with more confidence in a decision than each member would have alone (Janis 1982). Similarly, one researcher's confidence in a result may be buttressed by the confidence of a collaborator, which in turn is based partly on the confidence of the first researcher, so that confidence is more a function of group hysteria than of the validity of the result. Reliability may also suffer if one member of the team is weak but no one notices. There have been cases of scientific fraud in which one researcher fabricated data but the collaborators were strongly motivated to deny it (LaFollette 1992). As Hardwig (1985, 1991) has pointed out, we are very much epistemically dependent on one another: Much of what each of us professes to know depends on information that we have acquired from others whom we trust. The cost of epistemic dependence of the sort especially notable between collaborators is that mistakes can enter and propagate within the system because of collaborators who are inept or corrupt. Hence, collaboration between equals may both decrease and increase reliability.

In the Clearwater et al. experiment (1991) the different processors were virtually the same, but they developed varied approaches to a given cryptarithmetic problem because of the random generation of hypotheses. Similarly, even if two researchers are very similar, they will not pursue exactly the same solution to a problem because of subtle differences in what they know and in what they are exposed to. Collaboration can thus lead to increased power and speed as researchers working together produce more results in less time. There is no guarantee, of course. Loss of some power and speed in teacher-apprenticeship collaborations can be justified because of the long-term increase in fecundity that results from the training of a new researcher. With a peer-similar collaboration, it is an open question of whether progress justifies the time spent working together, but the collaborations mentioned earlier (Crick and Watson, Newell and Simon, Kahneman and Tversky) suggest that great progress can be made. Fecundity and efficiency (cost) do not seem to be issues for peer—similar collaborations.

It is important to recognize a relative difference between the kinds of results that may accrue from peer-similar collaborations compared with the first two kinds I discussed. Because employees and graduate students are more likely to be able to do the time-consuming routine work that experiments require than to make theoretical contributions, the gains associated with the first two kinds of collaboration are most likely to concern empirical results. In contrast, comparable collaborators have most to gain from each other conceptually, making progress toward theoretical results, although they can also benefit from working together to produce novel experimental designs. Molecular biologists frequently assist each other by using analogies between experiments: When a researcher's experiment is problematic, another researcher can describe a similar experiment that suggests a way of overcoming the problems (Dunbar 1995). Peer-different collaborations are even more strongly directed toward theoretical rather than empirical results.

In addition to those suggested by Goldman's epistemic standards, other reasons for collaboration may exist. Collaboration can be fun for reasons that are independent of power and speed. Having a collaborator can mean having someone you know is interested in discussing your research, thereby alleviating the loneliness of the long-distance scholar. Some researchers find it easier to develop new ideas in conversation rather than in individual thinking or writing. In addition, sociologists such as Latour (1987), who view science as an aggressive process of building alliances, might see collaborations a means of accumulating the political power to have one's ideas become dominant.

Enlisting collaborators is one way of increasing the competitiveness of one's research program (Durfee 1992). It is unlikely, however, that merely having a collaboration, as opposed to having a collaboration that produces good results, increases one's scientific success.

Peer—Different

Interdisciplinary fields such as cognitive science are the obvious places to look for collaborations among researchers with very different backgrounds. Here is a brief selection of cross-disciplinary collaborations in cognitive science, in alphabetical order:

- Robert Abelson (psychology) and Roger Schank (artificial intelligence)
- Patricia Churchland (philosophy) and Terry Sejnowski (computational neuroscience)
- Allan Collins (psychology) and M. R. Quinlan (artificial intelligence)
- Jerry Fodor (philosophy) and Zenon Pylyshyn (psychology)
- Ken Forbus (artificial intelligence) and Dedre Gentner (psychology)
- Kris Hammond (artificial intelligence) and Colleen Seifert (psychology)
- Geoffrey Hinton (artificial intelligence), Jay McClelland (psychology), David Rumelhart (psychology), and Paul Smolensky (physics, artificial intelligence)
- John Holland (artificial intelligence), Keith Holyoak (cognitive psychology), Richard Nisbett (social psychology), and Paul Thagard (philosophy, artificial intelligence)
- Mark Johnson (philosophy) and George Lakoff (linguistics)
- Daniel Osherson (psychology) and Scott Weinstein (philosophy)
- Michael Posner (psychology) and Marcus Raichle (neuroscience)

Schunn et al. (1995) surveyed papers presented at the annual meetings of the Cognitive Science Society and found a high frequency of interdisciplinary collaborations.

Because cross-disciplinary researchers use different methodologies (e.g., psychologists' experiments with human subjects versus artificial intelligence researchers' computer simulations), we should not expect empirical results to be the primary benefit of peer-different collaborations. But there are huge gains to be made in the number and rate of theoretical results. These gains in power and speed can come about because cross-disciplinary collaboration brings together previously isolated theoretical ideas that can produce fruitful combinations. Gains, however, are typically not the immediate result of cross-disciplinary work, since much time and effort must usually be expanded before people from different fields begin to understand each other. Peer-similar collaborators with the same kinds of intellectual background can expect to understand each other's work quickly, but extensive cross-disciplinary education is required for people from different fields to be able to work together productively. The time cost of interdisciplinary collaboration is illustrated by the fact that John Holland, Keith Holyoak, Richard Nisbett, and I spent more than a year meeting and talking regularly before we considered doing a book together (Holland, et al. 1986). Once intellectual barriers are overcome, however, there is a great potential gain in fecundity, since collaborative results can be developed and used by many people in many different fields.

Cross-disciplinary collaboration might contribute to reliability, through the triangulation of methods that lead to more robust results. An ideal cognitive science collaboration might be one that combined experiments on human behavior, computer simulations of that behavior, and brain scans of how that behavior is implemented in the human brain. The behavioral, computational, and neurological experiments would ideally provide a way of converging on valuable empirical and theoretical results. On the other hand, reliability can suffer from interdisciplinary collaboration if people from different fields have no way of critically evaluating the results of unfamiliar methodologies. Peer-different collaborators are exceptionally epistemically dependent on their coworkers, since they typically lack the skill to validate work conducted in a different field. Most psychologists, for example, know little about the pitfalls of computer modeling, just as most artificial intelligence researchers know little about the design of experiments that involve human subjects.

EXPLANATORY EFFICACY

Although Goldman's standards of reliability, power, speed, efficiency, and fecundity help us understand why cross-disciplinary collaboration can be a valuable epistemic strategy, they neglect an important aspect of scientific thought. The growth of scientific knowledge is not just a matter of the quantity and reliability of results: Some theoretical and empirical results are much more qualitatively important than others. Importance depends on the goals of inquiry. Scientists and other people do not strive simply to accumulate true beliefs. In everyday life, we want to acquire true beliefs relevant to our goals. In science, we want to acquire true beliefs that are relevant to the goals of science, which include explanation and technological application as well as truth. The greatest explanatory accomplishments of science are unifying theories, such as quantum theory and relativity theory in physics and evolutionary theory and genetics in biology. Cognitive science has not yet had its Newton,

Darwin, or Einstein to provide a unified theory that applies to all kinds of thinking, but many of the collaborations that have arisen in cognitive science have been important because of the steps they have provided toward theoretical unification.

A mature scientific field should not just be a list of unconnected results but rather unified by a common explanatory framework. Coherence is greatest when a few theoretical principles serve to explain many empirical observations. These principles, such as Darwin's central claim that species evolve as the result of natural selection, assume great importance because of their capacity to explain diverse observations. The observations increase in importance when they can be unified with others by means of the theory. Chapter 4 described how the bacterial theory of ulcers unifies numerous experimental observations.

Many collaborations in cognitive science, including both peer-similar and peer-different ones, derive their importance from the thrust toward unified theories. No single dominant theory has emerged, but collaborators have developed competing views of mind that have tied together diverse phenomena. For example, John Anderson (1983, 1993) and Allan Newell (1990) both have worked with many collaborators to show how diverse aspects of thinking can be viewed from the perspective of rule-based systems. Similarly, David Rumelhart and James McClelland (1986) both have worked with a host of collaborators to show the applicability of a different explanatory framework, parallel distributed processing.

Collaboration can increase explanatory coherence in two ways. First, collaboration, especially across disciplines, can produce conceptual combinations that establish new theoretical frameworks. Ideas about rule-based and artificial neural network systems have depended on integration of psychological and computational inspiration, as have ideas about analogical reasoning (Holyoak and Thagard 1995). Second, assembling a broad range of experimental results to be unified by a theoretical framework requires the participation of large groups of experimenters. Collaboration therefore greatly aids the production of unifying theories that have a demonstrably broad scope. Explanatory relations among the theoretical principles and the experimental results transform a set of independent results into a coherent whole (Thagard 1992b). Accordingly, I want to add the following to my version of Goldman's five standards:

> **6.** The *explanatory efficacy* of a practice is how well it contributes to the development of theoretical and experimental results that increase explanatory coherence.

To appreciate the practice of collaboration among researchers of equal stature, one must see how collaboration can be aimed at and can contribute to the explanatory efficacy of the results obtained. With this addition, Goldman's standards of social epistemic appraisal can shed considerable light on the advantages and disadvantages of collaboration in science. Chapter 12 discusses medicine's practical goal of improving patient health and also adds practical efficacy to the list of epistemic standards.

APPLICATIONS: ULCERS AND ANALOGY

The discussion so far has been programmatic and abstract, but it can easily be made more concrete by showing how the six standards for evaluating the benefits of collaboration apply in specific cases: (1) the bacterial theory of ulcers and (2) the multiconstraint theory of analogy.

Marshall and Warren: Ulcers

How did the collaboration among Barry Marshall, Robin Warren, and numerous colleagues rate according to the epistemic standards of reliability, power, fecundity, speed, efficiency, and explanatory efficacy? As described in chapter 6, collaboration was essential for the development of the bacterial theory of ulcers because of the involvement of several different medical specialties. Warren, a pathologist, noticed unusual spiral bacteria in gastric biopsies he examined in 1979, but he was unsure whether the bacteria had any medical significance. In 1981, he began working with Marshall, a trainee in gastroenterology. Together they devised an experiment that found an association between the bacteria and peptic ulcers. Subsequently, they were able to show that ulcers can often be cured by using antibiotics. In addition to Warren and Marshall's expertise in pathology and gastroenterology, the experiments required the know-how of specialists in microbiology, electron microsopy, and pharmacy. Marshall et al. (1988) has a total of nine coauthors drawn from four medical specialties.

It is obvious that Marshall could not have produced this important development on his own. As a gastroenterologist, he lacked the expertise to complete the pathology and microscopy work that was required to identify the presence of the bacteria. Similarly, Warren lacked the expertise to perform endoscopy to obtain the stomach biopsies. Having people other than experts use the instruments would have drastically reduced the reliability of the experimental results. The power and fecundity of collaboration is also evident, since Marshall and Warren acting without each other and without microbiologists and other assistants would never have been able to answer the question of whether *Helicobacter pylori* is a causal factor in ulcer disease. Speed and efficiency are lesser benefits of this collaboration, although it is clear that without a team of people to perform such tasks as biopsies, bacterial cultures, and statistical analyses, the research would have required much more time.

Collaboration can enhance explanatory efficacy in two ways: by contributing to theoretical and experimental results. The experimental results explained by the hypothesis that bacteria cause ulcers depended on collaboration. Although Marshall was responsible mainly for the formation and promulgation of this hypothesis, Warren contributed crucial links to Marshall's chain of reasoning, informing Marshall that the bacteria are associated with gastritis. When Marshall read that gastritis is associated with ulcers, he conjectured that the bacteria might be associated with ulcers (see chapter 3). Hence, collaboration contributed both theoretically and experimentally to explanatory coherence. In sum, the collaboration among Marshall, Warren, and their colleagues scores high on the standards of reliability, power, and explanatory efficacy.

Holyoak and Thagard: Analogy

In our 1995 book *Mental Leaps*, Keith Holyoak and I defended a theory of analogical thinking derived from more than a decade of collaborative work that combined Holyoak's expertise as an experimental psychologist and my background in philosophy and computational modeling. The preface of the book thanks more than thirty additional collaborators, including, for example, psychology graduate students who worked with Holyoak at Michigan and UCLA as well as programmers who worked with me at Princeton and Waterloo. Figure 11.4 summarizes some of the collaborations that made possible the theoretical, experimental, and computational work that went into our book.

Like many projects in cognitive science, this work combined several different methodologies that surpassed any individual's expertise. Whereas Holyoak and I worked jointly on theoretical issues, only he had the expertise to conduct rigorous psychological experiments, but he did not have sufficient computational background to write the computer programs that were essential to testing our theoretical claims against the psychological evidence. If Holyoak had tried to run the computer simulations, or if I had tried to conduct the psychological experiments, there would have been a dramatic loss in reliability. Instead, by combining experimental and computational skills, we were able to generate answers to many interesting questions concerning how people think analogically. It would be presumptuous to speak of the truth of our findings, but publication in respected journals such as *Cognitive Science* and *Artificial Intelligence* legitimates talk of results; hence, given my weakened version of Goldman's standards, we can say that our collaboration contributed to power and fecundity. The wealth of other collaborators also greatly enhanced the power of our research project, along with its speed and efficiency. In principle, Holyoak could have done all the experiments and I could have done all the simulations, but both enterprises are extremely time-consuming, and neither of us would have been able to do more than a fraction of what was eventually

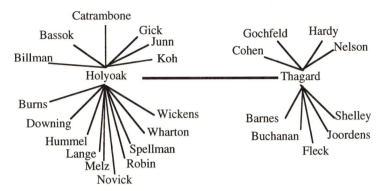

Figure 11.4. The collaborative nature of Holyoak and Thagard (1995). Names above Holyoak's are his Michigan collaborators; those below worked with him at the University of California, Los Angeles. Names above Thagard's are his Princeton collaborators; those below worked with him at Waterloo. All collaborators named were coauthors of published papers.

produced. Thus, experimental results, and the computational simulations that tied them with theory, were greatly fostered by collaboration.

Theoretical developments in this project were more narrowly collaborative, involving mostly Holyoak and me. Holyoak had the initial inspiration in 1987 that grew into our theory that analogical thinking fundamentally involves three kinds of constraints (structure, similarity, purpose). But subsequent theoretical contributions that emerged during the joint writing of numerous articles and the book are so entwined that it would be virtually impossible to disentangle them. Hence, on the presumption that it is legitimate to talk of theoretical and experimental results in this case, it is clear that explanatory efficacy was greatly aided by collaboration. As in the ulcers case, collaboration contributed to the development of the multiconstraint theory of analogy according to all six epistemic standards, but most notably power and explanatory efficacy.

The bacterial theory of ulcers, the multiconstraint theory of analogy, and innumerable theoretical and experimental results of current science show that scientific collaboration is a valuable social practice for promoting the development of scientific knowledge.

SUMMARY

Collaborative research is ubiquitous in the natural and social sciences, although it is still rare in the humanities. A scientist may collaborate with an employee, a student apprentice, a peer with similar background, or a peer with background in a different discipline. Different kinds of collaboration contribute in different ways to the reliability, power, fecundity, speed, efficiency, and explanatory efficacy of scientific research. The development of the bacterial theory of ulcers and of the multiconstraint theory of analogy illustrates the value of collaboration for advancing scientific knowledge.

CHAPTER 12

Medical Consensus

CHAPTER 6 described how the 1994 U.S. National Institutes of Health (NIH) Consensus Conference contributed to the widespread acceptance of the bacterial theory of ulcers. In the following three years, numerous other countries held similar conferences, and the American Digestive Health Foundation sponsored a second American consensus conference in February 1997. I attended the Canadian *Helicobacter pylori* Consensus Conference that took place in April 1997. This chapter begins with a description of the aims and events of the conference, but its main focus is on the following general question: How do medical consensus conferences contribute to medical knowledge and practice? After a discussion of the nature of evidence-based medicine and the logic involved in decisions about treatment and testing, I extend and apply Goldman's epistemic standards to evaluate the scientific and practical benefits of consensus conferences.

ANATOMY OF A CONSENSUS CONFERENCE

The Canadian *Helicobacter pylori* Consensus Conference was held in Ottawa on April 4 to 6, 1997, with sessions from Friday evening through Sunday morning. The eighty-one people in attendance included five jury members, twenty-one presenters, thirty-five participants, and twenty sponsors and supporters. The jury was given the prime responsibility for producing a report that summarized the best available treatments and tests for *H. pylori* infections. Members of the jury included John Bienenstock, an eminent clinical immunologist and former dean of the Faculty of Health Sciences at McMaster University, and other medical experts not directly involved in research on *H. pylori*. Most of the presenters, in contrast, had expertise in various aspects of *H. pylori* and related diseases. Many of the thirty-five participants who did not make presentations were practicing gastroenterologists involved in the treatment of peptic ulcers and related stomach problems. Also attending but not actively participating in the discussions were representatives of the sponsors of the conference, which included six pharmaceutical companies, two medical associations, and provincial governments.

The physical structure of the two full days of deliberations is indicated by figure 12.1, which is a diagram of how the people were seated in a large room.

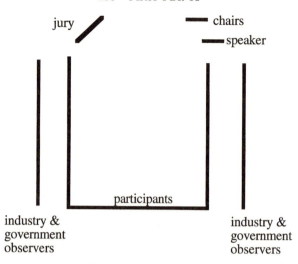

Figure 12.1. Seating of participants in the Canadian *Helicobacter pylori* Consensus Conference.

Notice that the five jury members were set off from the main participants (including presenters), as were the industry and government representatives. Although the pharmaceutical companies (Abbott, Astra, Axcan, Glaxo Wellcome, and Solvay) had paid the lion's share of the cost of the conference, it was clear from the start that they were expected to remain "at arm's length" from the discussions.

At the 1994 NIH consensus conference, the main question was whether peptic ulcers were caused by *H. pylori* and should be treated with antibiotics. Strikingly, at the 1997 Canadian conference, this was not even an issue; there was universal agreement that *H. pylori* is responsible for most peptic ulcers and that antibiotic treatment is appropriate. But the conference was charged with addressing numerous other issues important for the treatment of gastric disorders, including the following:

- Who should be tested for *H. pylori* infection and what tests should be used?
- Who should be treated for *H. pylori* infections?
- What are the most effective treatments for *H. pylori* infections?

The questions about testing and treatment of *H. pylori* would be much simpler if the bacteria were universally associated with disease. But as described in chapter 3, most people with *H. pylori* infections do not develop peptic ulcers, so it would be a great waste of medical resources to test everyone for the bacteria and give antibiotics to those found to be infected.

The most controversial issue at this conference was how to test and treat people with nonulcer dyspepsia (indigestion). According to conference presentations, dyspepsia occurs in twenty to forty percent of the population and is one of the major reasons for visits to physicians, after headache, backache, and fatigue. For dyspeptic patients with ulcers, testing and treatment for *H. pylori* infection was universally agreed to be appropriate, but the question for non-ulcer dyspepsia was more controversial. Whereas most patients with peptic ulcers have *H. pylori* infections whose eradication will cure the ulcers, the association between dyspepsia and *H. pylori* infection is much weaker. Hence, testing and treatment for *H. pylori* infection in patients who complain of indigestion is often unnecessary. Moreover, there are costs of different kinds for tests and treatments:

- Endoscopy (described in chapter 5) costs hundreds of dollars, is unpleasant, may have complications, and requires a patient to miss a day's work.
- Newer urea breath tests are not yet widely available in Canada, and one kind uses radioactive substances.
- Treatment with multiple antibiotics can be unpleasant and expensive.
- Widespread use of antibiotics can promote the spread of antibiotic-resistant strains of bacteria, rendering antibiotics ineffective when they are really needed.

The key issue, then, concerns what categories of patients should be tested and treated.

The conference addressed this and related issues through a series of presentations and discussions. On the first evening were talks on the basic mechanisms, epidemiology, and diagnosis of *H. pylori* infection. The Saturday sessions focused on treatment of *H. pylori* infection and included reports on new European and American guidelines, discussions of what disorders should be treated, and treatment in special populations such as children. Late Saturday afternoon, the conference divided into four workshops that were charged with discussing specific aspects of *H. pylori* treatment and testing. That evening there was a general dinner for the participants, but the jury attended a private dinner to discuss the day's presentations. On Sunday morning, there were lengthy reports from the workshop chairs, who presented the conclusions of their groups concerning such issues as when testing and treatment are appropriate. For each recommendation, there was discussion and a vote by all the participants, excluding representatives of industry and government. Unfortunately, these procedures took up the entire morning, so there was no time for the scheduled summary from the jury, which committed itself to distributing a report to all conference participants for further discussion. A draft report, containing the recommendations discussed later in this chapter, was mailed at the end of May, accompanied by a request for suggestions and comments to be sent to the conference organizers by mid-June. In July, the conference organizers mailed to all participants a substantially rewritten report, which was revised again and eventually published in the *Canadian Journal of Gastroenterology* (Hunt et al. 1998).

EVIDENCE-BASED MEDICINE

Several of the presenters at the Canadian consensus conference expressed a commitment to *evidence-based medicine*. This term initially struck me as internally redundant: What else could medicine be based on? But evidence-based medicine is an important movement in medical practice and pedagogy, in that it urges the "conscientious, explicit and judicious use of current best evidence in making decisions about the care of individual patients" (Sackett et al. 1996, p. 71). Carefully controlled clinical trials in medicine began only in 1948 and were rare until the 1960s (Bull 1959, Friedman et al. 1981). Only recently has medical education encouraged practicing physicians to consult the scientific literature directly for information about how best to treat patients.

Most practicing physicians have not been sufficiently trained in statistics and experimental design to be able to perform a stringent evaluation of the studies that are reported in the medical literature. Ideally, conclusions about the therapeutic value of different treatments should be based on randomized, double-blind experiments that track the results of interventions with minimal confounding variables (see chapter 5). The need for fully controlled experiments is clear from the account of causal reasoning that was summarized in Figure 7.2. To determine whether a treatment caused a patient to improve, we first need to determine whether patients given the treatment did better than ones not given the treatment—that is, whether $P(improvement/treatment) > P(improvement/no\ treatment)$. Hence the condition of patients given the treatment must be compared with that of a control group. But even if there is a difference between the treated group and the control group, we cannot infer that the treatment is causally effective, because the difference in improvement between the two groups might be due to some other factor. Members of the treated group may have been less ill than the control subjects such that their increased rate of improvement was not brought about by the treatment. However, when patients are randomly assigned to the treatment or control group, the experimenter has greater assurance that any difference found between the two groups is not the result of bias in allocation of patients or some other causally important difference between the groups. Similarly, double-blind studies, in which neither the patients nor the supervising clinicians know which subjects are in the treatment group versus the control group, are useful in ruling out the expectations of the patients and experimenters as spurious causes.

Unfortunately, randomized, double-blind, controlled trials in large populations are often so difficult and expensive to conduct that medical decisions must be based on weaker evidence. There is no established methodology or logic by which medical decision makers, whether members of consensus panels or practicing physicians, can translate the results of multiple clinical trials of varying quality into treatment recommendations. Mathematical decision theory, which recommends calculation of the expected utility of different actions using probabilities and numerical utilities of various outcomes, is rarely useful in this context. Calculation of the probability of improvement is not just a matter of taking a number from a clinical trial, because there may be different trials with different results and different designs. Meta-analysis is a statistical technique that provides a way of combining the data from different studies, but it presupposes that the studies combined all are methodologically adequate.

Because the evidence showing that antibiotics cured peptic ulcers was strong by 1997, there was no need for participants at the conference to worry greatly about the quality of particular trials. However, several presenters remarked on the equivocal nature of the evidence concerning the effectiveness of treating dyspepsia by eradicating *H. pylori*. Nevertheless, there was much deliberation that concerned testing for and treating *H. pylori* in dyspepsia patients.

THE LOGIC OF TESTING AND TREATMENT

Discussions of testing and treatment at the conference, like all real-life arguments, were fluid and diverse. It was clear that there is no formalized logic for making decisions on medical policy. Issues about who and how to test and who and how to treat do not reduce to any neat algebraic cost-benefit analysis. I was not the only participant at the conference who was struggling with difficult decisions such as whether to test and treat people with nonulcer dyspepsia. I was, perhaps, the only participant who was struggling to understand the *logic* of the decisions, which concerns how medical experts do and should bring scientific evidence to bear on questions that concern testing treatment.

At a highly general level, the decisions that were the subject of this conference can be understood in terms a model of deliberative coherence that is analogous to the model of explanatory coherence that was applied to theory evaluation in chapter 4 (see Millgram and Thagard 1996; Thagard and Millgram 1995). Whereas theory evaluation and causal reasoning involve assessing the coherence of hypotheses with respect to the evidence and each other, deliberative coherence involve assessing the coherence of actions with respect

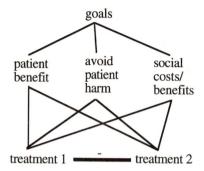

Figure 12.2. Medical decision as a coherence problem. Thin lines indicate positive constraints that specify, for example, the extent to which treatment 1 benefits patients. The thick line is a negative constraint indicating that two treatments are incompatible.

to different goals. Figure 12.2 shows very roughly how this interaction works in a decision concerning what treatments to adopt. It depicts a decision between two treatments (one of which might be to do nothing), taking into account the goals of helping patients, avoiding harm to patients, and avoiding social costs such as unnecessary healthcare expenditures. Unspecified in the figure, and in most real-life deliberations, are the relative priorities of these three goals, as well as the extent to which the various goals are facilitated by the different treatments available. The question of relative priorities of goals is a question for ethics rather than medical research, although the latter should be the source of information about the contributions of different treatments to different goals.

Unfortunately, the complexity of medical research makes it difficult to plug in a value for the extent to which a treatment produces benefits. What should a consensus jury do when evidence is equivocal, as it is concerning the benefits of *H. pylori* eradication for patients with dyspepsia? At its meeting in September 1996, the European *Helicobacter pylori* Study Group based its recommendations for treating different conditions on three categories of scientific evidence: unequivocal(1) supportive(2) and equivocal(3) (Malfertheiner et al. 1997). Similarly, the recommendations for treatment of *H. pylori* infection were graded in three categories: strongly recommended(A) advisable(B) and uncertain(C). However, there was no simple one-to-one mapping between their levels of evidence and their recommendations, as is shown in Table 12.1.

It seems odd that the European study group gave a "2. Advisable" recommendation for functional dyspepsia based on a "3. Equivocal" assessment of the scientific evidence. They gave the rationale that, although the scientific evidence for the improvement of the actual symptoms after *H. pylori* eradication is lacking, the expected benefit on the gastritis status makes it advisable to

TABLE 12.1

European Recommendations for *Helicobacter pylori*
Eradication in Different Clinical Conditions

Disease	Recommendation (overall evaluation)	Scientific Evidence
DU/GU (active or not)	1	A
MALToma	1	A
Gastritis with severe abnormalities	1	B
Post early gastric cancer resection	1	B
Functional dyspepsia	2	C
Family history of gastric cancer	2	C
GERD	2	B
NSAID therapy	2	C
Post surgery for PUD	2	B
Asymptomatic subjects	3	C
Extra-alimentary tract diseases	3	C

Source: From a handout distributed at the Canadian *Helicobacter pylori* Consensus Conference. DU/GU, duodenal ulcer or gastric ulcer; GERD, gastroesophageal reflux disease; MALToma, mucosa-assisted lymphoid tissue lymphoma; NSAID, nonsteroidal anti-inflammatory drug; PUD, peptic ulcer disease.

eradicate *H. pylori* after full investigation to exclude organic disorders. The reasoning here seems to be this: We can't really say whether eradicating patients' bacteria will help their dyspepsia, but it will at least eliminate their gastritis and possibly reduce their long-term risk of peptic ulcers and gastric cancer. The cogency of this reasoning is not overwhelming.

The U.S. consensus conference that took place in February 1997 was more cautious. Sponsored by the American Digestive Health Foundation, this update conference was organized in a format similar to that of the 1994 NIH Consensus Development Conference, with a multidisciplinary panel reviewing presentations from international experts. Like the European group, this panel recommended *H. pylori* testing and treatment for duodenal ulcer, gastric ulcer, gastric ulcer, and MALT (mucosa-assisted lymphoid tissue) lymphoma. But the panel made no recommendation for the universal testing of patients with dyspepsia, concluding that testing for and treating such patients for *H. pylori* infection has not been adequately investigated in terms of effectiveness, symptom relief, patient satisfaction, and cost (Peura et al. in press). The panel recommended the performance of well-designed clinical trials to assess the impact of *H. pylori* testing and treatment on patients with dyspepsia.

At the Canadian conference, the workshop that discussed treatment similarly concluded that there should be no general recommendation concerning dyspepsia, but it proposed that *H. pylori* testing and treatment could be appropriate on an individual basis. The May 1997 draft and the final report recommended that patients with chronic dyspepsia and persistent and/or frequent symptoms be considered on a case-by-case basis for noninvasive (testing e.g., serology or urea breath test) and subsequent treatment. Like the European study, the concern seemed to be that some of the dyspepsia patients were at risk of acquiring ulcers. Notably, neither the U.S. panel nor the Canadian workshop made a recommendation *against* testing and treating dyspeptic patients. Unlike the European conference, the Canadian and U.S. conferences did not recommend testing and treatment for gastroesophageal reflux disease. A speaker at the Canadian conference reported that the European conclusion was based on a 1996 study in the *New England Journal of Medicine* that was poorly controlled and not replicated by new, as yet unpublished trials.

Unlike the question of who to treat for *H. pylori* infection, the question of how to treat them can be answered very satisfactorily. The European, Canadian, and U.S. consensus conferences all noted the availability of several combination drug treatments that successfully eradicate the bacteria in more than eighty percent of patients. Physicians can then choose among these on the basis of cost and ease of compliance.

Testing raises issues similar to those concerned with treatment: Who should be tested, and what tests should be used? Similar issues arise with other diseases, for example, when mammograms should be used as a screening test for breast cancer, and when prostate-specific antigen (PSA) tests should be used to screen for prostate cancer. The American Cancer Society recommends a PSA test in all men older than fifty years, but the test has numerous drawbacks. Of every one hundred men older than fifty years, testing finds ten with elevated PSA levels, but only three of these will actually have prostate cancer (see http://www.ices.on.ca/docs/fb1290.htm). Hence, seven out of one hundred men will unnecessarily undergo the anxiety of possibly having cancer and the unpleasantness of procedures such as needle biopsies. The risk of these unnecessary treatments would be worthwhile if early detection in the three men who are found to have prostate cancer actually saved lives, but many prostate cancers are slow growing, and there is little evidence that early detection by PSA screening reduces death rates. Moreover, treatment of prostate cancer by surgery or radiation often has side effects such as incontinence and impotence. Hence, it is not at all obvious that there are grounds for the general use of the PSA test (see also Middleton 1997). A fifty-year-old man with no prostate symptoms may be more likely to derive stress, unnecessary procedures, and treatment side effects from taking a PSA test than to derive increased longevity.

In women older than fifty years, mammograms have been found effective in detecting breast cancers sufficiently early that prognosis is improved, but no similar effect has been found for mammograms in younger women. A test is now available to determine whether a woman carries mutations in the BRCA1 gene that disposes them toward breast cancer, but medical knowledge is insufficient to advise a response to this information. Deciding whether to test requires careful examination of the costs and benefits of obtaining the different results of the test. Physicians often use the age of thirty-five years as a basis for advising a pregnant woman to have amniocentesis to screen for birth defects, because at this age the probability of having a retarded child becomes equal to the probability of having a miscarriage induced by the procedure. Obviously, however, different families have very different evaluations of the effects of a miscarriage versus the effects of raising a retarded child.

At the Canadian *Helicobacter pylori* Consensus Conference, there was general agreement against testing of asymptomatic individuals. It is unreasonable to test all thirty million Canadians, because most of the seven million believed to be infected with *H. pylori* bacteria will not suffer disease as a result. In contrast, if a patient has ulcer symptoms such as burning pain in the upper abdomen, testing for *H. pylori* is clearly desirable, since eradicating the bacteria will likely produce a cure. But what should a physician do with a patient with dyspepsia who may have found out about *H. pylori* on television or the World Wide Web? There is no point in having the patient tested unless the physician intends to treat the patient with antibiotics; we have already seen that there is no clear evidence that eradicating the bacteria helps much with dyspepsia. On the other hand, if the physician refuses to order the test, the patient is likely to be upset and find another physician who is more compliant. The physician might also fear legal action if the patient is not tested but turns out to have a serious condition such as gastric cancer. In the end, the Canadian consensus conference left it up to individual physicians to decide whether a dyspeptic patient should be tested for *H. pylori*. Blood tests and urea tests are relatively reliable and much less invasive than endoscopy, so they are the preferred response to the question of how to test.

CONTRIBUTIONS OF CONSENSUS CONFERENCES

What are the intended and actual contributions of consensus conferences to the growth of medical knowledge? Chapter 11 assessed scientific collaboration with respect to six epistemic standards: reliability, power, fecundity, speed, efficiency, and explanatory efficacy. All these standards are concerned with theoretical results and ignore the practical aims of applied science. Although much medical research is basic and theoretical, its ultimate aim is to improve health. Consensus conferences are held to improve patient care, not just to help settle theoretical disputes. Hence, understanding of consensus conferences requires consideration of an additional standard:

7. The *pragmatic efficacy* of a practice is how well it leads to the accomplishment of goals such as human welfare.

For medical practices such as consensus conferences, the key goal is human health. Usually, satisfaction of epistemic standards such as reliability and explanatory efficacy contributes to pragmatic efficacy, because medical treatments based on evidence are usually much more effective in promoting human health than are those with no empirical support. But the last section showed that the relation of evidence to medical recommendations is not at all simple, and consensus conferences need to help the medical profession extract practical lessons about testing and treatment. Accordingly, I assess the intended pragmatic efficacy of consensus conferences after discussing them in terms of the six epistemic standards. I use the veritistic (truth-related) versions of Goldman's standards rather than the results-related standards used in chapter 11, which were concerned with explaining the relatively short-term decisions of whether scientists should collaborate. The assessment of medical conferences is made from a more long-term perspective.

Reliability and Explanatory Efficacy

There are a number of ways that medical consensus conferences foster the reliability of medical research, that is, the ratio of truths to the total number of beliefs produced. There are many forces that can impede medical reliability, including the following:

- Some medical researchers have personal ambitions such as fame and financial interests that may cloud their assessment of evidence.
- Some medical practitioners have financial and professional incentives to use some treatments rather than others.
- Some pharmaceutical companies that fund research are motivated to increase profits.

Ideally, a medical consensus conference should be structured to ignore these interests and make decisions based on evidence and benefit to patients.

Consensus conferences such as the one I attended and the ones sponsored by the NIH are structured to increase the reliability of their conclusions. First, they bring together numerous experts from various medical fields. Presenters at the Canadian *Helicobacter pylori* Consensus Conference included epidemiologists and infectious disease specialists as well as gastroenterologists from several countries. No one person could be expected to be fully expert in all the fields relevant to decisions concerning the treatment of ulcers and dyspepsia, so the conference served the function of bringing together information from numerous sources. Of course, having multiple presenters would be useless if they lacked the credentials and knowledge to justify reliance on their presentations, but the organizers of consensus conferences choose carefully whom they invite. Researchers on the cutting edge of their fields can often report research that is in press or in progress rather than only what has been published.

Second, consensus conferences encourage discussion and dissent among the participants. Experts do not always agree, and listening to their arguments can be an effective way for a disinterested observer to get a balanced perspective on contentious issues. At the Canadian conference, workshops provided the opportunity for discussion in smaller groups, supplementing the occasionally lively arguments that took place in the full sessions. All the participants were encouraged to make suggestions and comments on the draft document distributed after the conference.

Third, the reliability of the conclusions of consensus conferences it encouraged by the presence of an independent jury. Jury members are selected from medical personnel and others with no personal stake in the decision to be made. Because they have no financial or professional interest in particular outcomes, they can impartially judge the evidence and arguments presented to them. At the 1994 NIH Consensus Conference on ulcers, some presenters, such as Marshall, obviously had a personal interest in seeing their ideas endorsed by the panel, but the panel itself was initially neutral on the issues it evaluated.

Fourth, consensus conferences exclude from decision making the representatives of pharmaceutical companies and other agencies with a clear interest that may conflict with reliability. The selection of the presenters and the jury members ensures the exclusion of drug companies' concerns about the profitability of their products and healthcare organizations' concerns about minimizing costs. The seating plan of the Canadian conference shown in Figure 12.1, which separated the representatives of industry and government from the main participants, was intended to reinforce the aim of the conference to make decisions on the basis of evidence rather than the lobbying of interest groups.

In sum, medical consensus conferences are social processes that seem well designed to promote the reliability of conclusions. Like any other cognitive and social process, they are fallible and may not succeed in producing correct results. Even though they are structured to diminish the effects of epistemically illegitimate interests, the nature of the human participants cannot be expected to be completely eliminated. At the Canadian, European, and U.S. consensus conferences, there was some pressure to legitimate the use of *H. pylori* eradication for dyspepsia, even though the evidence for its effectiveness was equivocal. Practicing gastroenterologists clearly had the worry that if they did not treat a dyspeptic patient with antibiotics to eradicate *H. pylori*, the patient would quickly find someone else who would. It is possible that for some participants the desire to retain patients was a factor that went beyond and perhaps interfered with the official "evidence-based" approach of the conference.

Because the conference was concerned with the evaluation of existing hypotheses rather than the production of new explanatory theories and explained evidence, the standard of explanatory efficacy in this case was basically the same as reliability, so no additional discussion of it is necessary.

Power and Fecundity

In Goldman's (1992) epistemic standards, the power of a practice is its ability to produce true answers to questions of interest, and the fecundity of a practice is its ability to lead to large number of true beliefs for *many* practitioners. Medical consensus conferences, unlike medical researchers, do not generate answers that are absolutely new, but their conclusions are often new for some of the participants and especially for the larger audience for whom the deliberations are intended. The aim of a consensus conference is not simply to increase the knowledge of the participants but, more important, to increase knowledge throughout the medical community. The conclusions of these conferences are typically promulgated in medical journals and sometimes in the popular media. The need for such promulgation is evident in Figure 12.3, which shows the discrepancy in 1994 between gastroenterologists and primary physicians in their use of *H. pylori* eradication. Whereas ninety-nine percent of specialists responding to the survey had used this treatment, only sixty-four percent of primary physicians had. The results of a broader 1995 survey by Munnangi and Sonnenberg (1997) were even more striking: Only five percent of patients were receiving antibiotic therapy. Consensus conferences increase the spread of reliable knowledge by first instructing the participants of the conferences and then providing reports of the conferences recommendations to the full audience of people who are reached by the media.

I was initially puzzled as to why there was a need for a *Canadian* consensus conference in addition to the U.S. and European conferences. One reason that consensus conferences need to be organized nationally is that the lines of communication are often national. Canadian physicians are likely eventually to hear of new medical breakthroughs through their own journals, such as the *Canadian Journal of Gastroenterology* and the *Canadian Medical Association Journal*. Another reason is that different countries have different populations at risk for various diseases: In Canada, *H. pylori* infection and resulting gastric problems are much more common among Aboriginal natives and recent immigrants from Asia, two groups that are relatively larger in Canada than in the United States. Finally, practical decisions about tests and treatments are in part economic issues, and the economics of healthcare differ dramatically among countries. In Canada's national health system, the government pays for most health costs, whereas in the United States payment is made primarily through

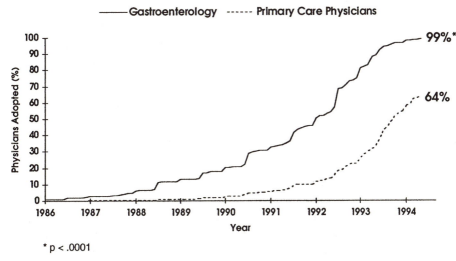

Figure 12.3. Adoption of *Helicobacter pylori* eradication therapy and the timing of first use by specialty. *p < .0001 From Fendrick et al. (1996, p. 1547). Reprinted with permission from the American College of Gastroenterology.

a multitude of private insurance companies. Canada also differs from the United States in having more patients treated by primary physicians, with less access to specialists.

Speed and Efficiency

Consensus conferences are expensive, in that they require the transporting, housing, and feeding of numerous participants. But a three-day conference is a relatively rapid means of exchanging information, establishing recommendations, and providing the basis for spreading reliable conclusions to a broad audience. Clarfield et al. (1996) studied a consensus conference on dementia and found that the information presented influenced attendees to change their initial recommendations. In the absence of other obvious social process for establishing and communicating evidence-based conclusions, the medical consensus conference seems to fare well on the standards of speed and efficiency.

Pragmatic Efficacy

Ultimately, the standard by which medical consensus conferences must be evaluated is how successful they are in improving the effectiveness of healthcare. Do patients receive better treatment as the result of consensus conferences? There is no direct way of answering the question, but it would seem that the reliability and fecundity of the conferences should translate into better healthcare. Physicians and hospitals can learn not only from the treatments recommended by consensus panels but also learn from the treatments *not* recommended: Consensus statements provide health care providers with reasons *not* to give ineffective treatments to people who may be requesting them based on weak information. Today's patients may march into their physicians' offices with a printout from the World Wide Web in their hands, but there is great variability in the quality of such information (see chapter 13). Evidence-based and cost-effective medicine instituted through the recommendations of consensus conferences should improve patient care.

Evidence-based medical consensus conferences provide an excellent illustration of how social processes of communication and discussion can interact with individual cognitive processes of explanatory coherence. Participants may arrive at the conference with different causal beliefs based on different evidence and hypotheses. Through discussion, however, the full range of evidence and explanations can become available to all participants. Then, by assessing the explanatory coherence of competing hypotheses with respect to all the evidence, the conference participants can reach a consensus that is publicized to a wider audience.

SUMMARY

Scientific consensus arises from social processes of communication and persuasion. In medicine, the development of consensus is facilitated by the holding of conferences that are designed to make recommendations for improving patient care. These recommendations are evidence based, drawing whenever possible on the results of randomized, controlled clinical trials that assess the effectiveness of various treatments. Decisions about treatment and testing are often difficult, because of conflicting evidence and the complexity of assessing the consequences of different medical practices. By virtue of their use of expert testimony and impartial panels, medical consensus conferences can contribute to the reliability, fecundity, and practical benefit of medical beliefs.

CHAPTER 13

Science and Medicine on the Internet

CONSENSUS CONFERENCES and collaboration are social processes that encourage the development of medical knowledge. During the 1990s, new technologies have brought about dramatic changes in the way science is conducted, thereby transforming communication and collaboration. Internet technologies, including electronic mail, preprint archives, and the World Wide Web, are now ubiquitous parts of scientific and medical practice. After reviewing the full range of these technologies and sketching the history of their development, this chapter provides an appraisal of their contributions to scientific research. It again uses Alvin Goldman's epistemic criteria of reliability, power, fecundity, speed, and efficiency to evaluate the largely positive impact of Internet technologies on the development of scientific knowledge.

A DAY IN THE LIFE OF A CYBERSCIENTIST

Here is how a work day unfolds for a scientist who makes use of the full range of Internet technologies. Consider an imaginary scientist, Marie Darwin, who works in a field such as biomedicine or physics, for which the Internet provides many resources. She arrives at work in the morning and immediately checks her electronic mail (e-mail), finding that she has numerous messages. Some of these are from her students, asking for advice on how to run the experiments they are planning, and she responds with technical instructions that they can read the next time they check their own e-mail. Another message is from Charles Curie, a collaborator of Marie's working at another research institute in a different country, who has some ideas for developing the new theory that he and Marie are trying to construct to explain their experimental results. Marie responds with some improvements to Charles's hypotheses, and she e-mails him a first draft of a paper she is writing in collaboration with him, so that he can revise it and e-mail a second draft back to her. In addition, Marie has e-mail from a journal editor telling her that her most recent paper is accepted if she is willing to make a few changes suggested by referees who e-mailed their reviews to the editor.

Marie now accesses the World Wide Web, first checking her local institute Web page for news about visiting speakers. More important to her research, she links to the preprint archive for her field, which contains electronic versions of papers not yet published. Marie is quickly able to see that ten new papers in her special area of research have been posted to the archive since the previous day. She clicks on the names of the papers to read the summaries and makes a note to download several of them for more thorough examination later. Marie then sends a new paper that she finished the day before to the preprint archive, knowing that it will be quickly available to all the other researchers working on similar topics. Now she is ready to use the Web for her ongoing research.

Marie begins her most important work of the day by using a Web link to an internal site at her institute that is accessible to her research group. Immediately, she can see that her students and research assistants working late the previous night have collected some new experimental data that she examines on her screen. These data raise a question about similar observations made in Charles's laboratory, so she finds the link to that lab's Web site and goes into a database that contains the results of their experiments from the previous year. To find the particular data that interest her, she uses a search engine that Charles's lab has provided to take her immediately to the part of the large database that contains the information she wants.

This information, along with the new experimental results from her own lab, raise some interesting questions concerning the structure of the objects that she and Charles are investigating. Fortunately, another research institute has provided a Web site that vividly displays what is known about such structures, so she moves to that site and uses a search engine to call up the relevant objects. There, she can examine their structure using several valuable tools that go well beyond the presentation of the simple two-dimensional pictures that are found in textbooks. She first runs a special Virtual Reality browser to examine three-dimensional representations of the objects, using her mouse to navigate through the representation to view the objects from different angles. She then downloads an animation that enables her to watch the objects moving together over time. Together, the animation and the three-dimensional model suggest a new theoretical insight into how these objects might produce the experimental effects that she has been finding in her work. Because testing her new theoretical ideas requires some new software that has just become available for interpreting the kind of data she has collected, Marie follows a link to another Web site that makes the software available. She is pleased to see that she does not have to download the software but can immediately run the program on her own computer as a Java application that is automatically set up for her by her Web browser. Excited by what the program suggests about her data, she e-mails Charles and her students a sketch of her new ideas and results, suggesting a time when they can have a collective Web conference during which they can interactively discuss new research directions.

The story I have just told is not speculative science fiction: Every technology it mentions is currently available on the Internet and is in use by scientists, although of course not all scientists use every technology. The Internet, particularly the World Wide Web, is now an essential part of scientific communication. By examining the ways that scientists are now using these resources to further the development of scientific research, we can see how new technologies can contribute to the spread of knowledge.

REVOLUTIONS IN SCIENTIFIC COMMUNICATION

In the 1450s, Johann Gutenberg used his new invention of the printing press to produce hundreds of copies of the Bible. In the following century, the printing of books had a dramatic influence on the development of scientific knowledge (Eisenstein 1979, Vol. 2). The printing and distribution of astronomical observations contributed to the downfall of Claudins Ptolemy's theory that the sun revolved around the earth. Nicolaus Copernicus and others noticed discrepancies between the predictions of Ptolemy's theory and actual observations, and they constructed an alternative theory that placed the sun at the center of the planetary system. Similarly, widespread publication of books on Galen's anatomy brought into question the accuracy of his descriptions of the human body, leading Andreas Vesalius and others to produce and publish more accurate depictions. The first scientific journals were started in 1665 and provided a means for scholars to communicate their findings that was far more efficient than the personal letters used previously.

In the 1990s, communication underwent another dramatic revolution with the development of the World Wide Web and other Internet applications. Conceived in the 1960s as a U.S. military communications system called the ARPANET, the Internet became in the 1980s a convenient means of scientific communication, enabling scientists at major research institutions to send e-mail, participate in news groups, and transfer files. Working at the European particle physics laboratory CERN, in 1989 Tim Berners-Lee proposed a networked project for high-energy physics collaborations, employing hypertext to provide a flexible means of linking words and pictures. By 1991, his group had produced a simple browser for their "World Wide Web" project, which was superseded in 1993 by a more sophisticated browser, Mosaic, produced in the United States by the National Center for Supercomputer Applications (NCSA). Mosaic was in turn quickly supplanted by more sophisticated browsers such as Netscape Navigator and Internet Explorer. The number of hosts on the Internet grew from 213 in 1981 to 313,000 in 1990, then to more than twenty-nine million in 1998; the number of Web sites grew from 130 in mid-1993 to an estimated 650,000 in 1997. (This information is due to Network Wizards, available at http://www.nw.com/; and to Matthew Gray of the Massachusetts Institute of Technology [MIT], at http://www.mit.edu/people/ mkgray/net. Historical information about the Internet is available on the Web, e.g., at http://www.cern.ch/CERN/WorldWideWeb/RCTalk/history.html.)

These tools have inspired thousands of scientists to create Web sites and Internet tools that are dramatically changing how science is done. To show how the Internet is transforming scientific research practices, I describe how the Web is used at CERN, where it was first invented, as well as how it makes possible rapid and effective communication in the Human Genome Project and other research. Like the application of the printing press to scientific publishing, use of the World Wide Web has enabled scientists to increase the reliability, speed, and efficiency of their work.

SCIENCE ON THE WEB

By the end of 1996, the Internet guide Yahoo! listed more than a thousand Web sites each for astronomy, biology, earth sciences, and physics, along with many hundreds of sites for other sciences, such as chemistry and psychology (available at http://www.yahoo.com/Science/). Although many of these sites are used to provide general information to scientists and the public, some sites have become integral to research activities. In 1991, Paul Ginsparg, a physicist at the Lost Alamos National Library, created a database of new physics papers. By 1996, this archive served more than thirty-five thousand users from over seventy countries, with seventy-thousand electronic transactions per day. Physicists daily use the World Wide Web to check for newly written and as yet unpublished papers in their research areas. (A paper by Ginsparg is available at http://xxx.lanl.gov/blurb/pg96unesco.html. The physics preprint site is at http://xxx.lanl.gov:80/.)

The Web has also become a regular tool used by many scientists in the production of their research. Especially in fields such as high-energy physics and genetics, contemporary science is a huge collaborative enterprise that involves international teams of scientists (see chapter 12). It is not unusual for published articles in physics to have more than a hundred coauthors, reflecting the diversity of expertise needed to carry out large projects that involve complex instruments. Located near Geneva, CERN is a collaborative project of nineteen European countries that involves several nuclear accelerators and dozens of experimental research projects. Each project involves numerous different researchers from a range of different institutions in the participating counties. Since it began in 1954, CERN has been the source of many of the most important discoveries in particle physics, such as the 1983 finding of evidence for the top quark.

The World Wide Web was invented at CERN to improve information sharing among scientists from diverse institutions working on joint projects. It was conceived as a hypermedia project so that scientists could exchange pictorial information such as diagrams and data graphs as well as verbal text. Today, CERN has a World Wide Web team to support experiments, using a total of about 160 Web servers (available at http://www.cern.ch/).

The basic idea of the World Wide Web originated in a document written in 1989 by Tim Berners-Lee (available at http://www.w3.org/pub/WWW/History/1989/proposal.html). He argued as follows:

> CERN is a wonderful organisation. It involves several thousand people, many of them very creative, all working toward common goals. Although they are nominally organized into a hierarchical management structure, this does not constrain the way people will communicate, and share information, equipment and software across groups.
>
> The actual observed working structure of the organisation is a multiply connected "web" whose interconnections evolve with time. In this environment, a new person arriving, or someone taking on a new task, is normally given a few hints as to who would be useful people to talk to. Information about what facilities exist and how to find out about them travels in the corridor gossip and occasional newsletters, and the details about what is required to be done spread in a similar way. All things considered, the result is remarkably successful, despite occasional misunderstandings and duplicated effort.
>
> A problem, however, is the high turnover of people. When two years is a typical length of stay, information is constantly being lost. The introduction of the new people demands a fair amount of their time and that of others before they have any idea of what goes on. The technical details of past projects are sometimes lost forever, or only recovered after a detective investigation in an emergency. Often, the information has been recorded, it just cannot be found.
>
> If a CERN experiment were a static once-only development, all the information could be written in a big book. As it is, CERN is constantly changing as new ideas are produced, as new technology becomes available, and in order to get around unforeseen technical problems. When a change is necessary, it normally affects only a small part of the organisation. A local reason arises for changing a part of the experiment or detector. At this point, one has to dig around to find out what other parts and people will be affected. Keeping a book up to date becomes impractical, and the structure of the book needs to be constantly revised.

Berners-Lee recommended that the information at CERN should be handled not as a linear book or a hierarchical tree, but as hypertext. He had previous experience with hypertext, having in 1980 written a program for keeping track of software that he later adapted for use at CERN. He outlined how CERN could benefit from a large noncentralized hypermedia system, linking graphics, speech, video, and text in an unconstrained way that would enable users to jump from one entry to another. He stated that researchers needed remote access for the many computers used at CERN, independent of the particular kind of computer used. Berners-Lee presciently noted that CERN's diverse computer network was a miniature of the world in a few years' time, anticipating that the World Wide Web would not merely be a local application.

CERN's various research groups now make extensive use of the World Wide Web. For example, the DELPHI (DEtector for Lepton, Photon and Hadron Identification) project at CERN involves about 550 physicists from fifty-six participating universities and institutes in twenty-two countries (available at http://www.cern.ch/Delphi/Welcome.html). These scientists can use the Web to access data acquired over the past eight years, including pictorial representations of important experimental events. Also available are DELPHI news bulletins, a discussion forum, and electronic versions of papers by the projects' participants as well as links to preprint servers, participating institutions, and other physics information sources.

After CERN's programmers initiated use of the World Wide Web for scientific research, they made the software they had developed freely available, and international Web use expanded rapidly with the development of more sophisticated browsers. One of the most effective scientific users of the Web has been the Human Genome Project, an international consortium of research institutions working since 1989 to identify all the approximately 100,000 genes that are responsible for human development. This project is medically important, because many diseases such as diabetes and some forms of cancer have a large genetic component. The identification of all human genes should be a substantial aid to finding genes responsible for diseases, which can potentially lead to new medical treatments.

Scientists working on the genome project are producing an astonishing amount of information. If published in books, descriptions of the DNA sequences of all the human genes would require more than 200,000 pages (available at http://www.ornl.gov/TechResources/Human_Genome/publicat/primer/intro.html). However, books would be a poor technology for keeping track of such information, not just because of the quantity of information, but also because new genes are being mapped daily and a printed text would be instantly obsolete. Fortunately, genome scientists have turned to computer databases to store the rapidly expanding information about gene locations. Storing this information would be useless, however, without effective means for accessing it, which search engines provide. Like CERN, the Human Genome Project is highly collaborative, involving dozens of different institutions in various countries. The arrival of the World Wide Web has been an immense boon to international collaboration on the genome project, with more than twenty-five contributing institutions making their data available on the Web for general access.

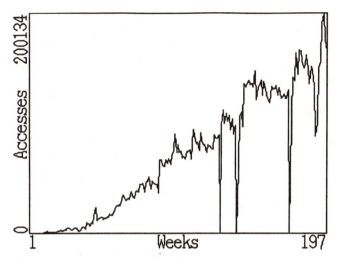

Figure 13.1. Web site accesses at the Massachusetts Institute of Technology Human Genome Center from May 1994 to February 1998. From http://www-genome.wi.mit.edu/www/usage/index.html. Reproduced by permission.

One of the major contributors to the genome project is the Human Genome Center at the Whitehead Institute at MIT (available at http://www-genome.wi.mit.edu/). Since its creation in May 1994, the number of weekly accesses to their Web site has grown to more than 200,000 (Figure 13.1). Internal users from MIT and external users from various institutions access the gene mapping information as well as various documents and software that are available at the site. Like other genome project sites, the MIT site contains searchable databases that researchers can consult to find the latest information.

For medical researchers, a more directly useful database is Online Mendelian Inheritance in Man (OMIM), available since December 1995 (http://www3.ncbi.nlm.nih.gov/Omim/). The reference book Mendelian Inheritance in Man (eleventh edition, McKusick and Francomano 1994) has been a valuable source of information on genetic traits and diseases, but the World Wide Web version is even more useful. Whereas the reference book was updated approximately every two years, OMIM is updated almost daily. It has an excellent search engine that enables users to quickly access entries about characters, genes, and diseases, and the entries provide links to relevant information such as genome maps and journal references. Whereas the reference book is expensive ($165) and typically found only in research libraries, anyone with Internet access can quickly obtain the information available on OMIM.

CERN, the Human Genome Project, and OMIM illustrate only some of the technologies available to scientists over the World Wide Web (Renehan 1996). Various sites provide animations and videos that enable viewers to see nature in motion. The Virtual Reality Modeling Language is beginning to be used to enable scientists to view objects in three dimensions, for example, in the Image Library of Biological Macromolecules (available at http://www.vrml.org/ and http://www.imb-jena.de/IMAGE.html). A different kind of virtual reality environment is AstroVR, a multiuser networked environment with access to many astronomical tools and databases (available at http://brando.ipac.caltech.edu:8888/). It enables astronomers and astrophysicists equipped with the proper software and hardware to talk, work together on a whiteboard, share images, make data plots, and look up astronomical data and literature. The goal of AstroVR is to enable users to interact and do collaborative research almost as if they were in the same room. Sites such as the NCSA Biology Workbench make computer programs and other tools readily available to scientific researchers (http://biology.ncsa.uiuc.edu/).

EVALUATION OF THE INTERNET ACCORDING TO EPISTEMIC CRITERIA

These exciting scientific uses of the World Wide Web provide examples of how it is contributing to the development of knowledge. To examine this contribution more comprehensively, we can use Goldman's veritistic standards of reliability, power, fecundity, speed, and efficiency to evaluate how well different social practices lead to true beliefs. I show how each of these standards enables us to see more clearly why the printing press was so important for communication, and I apply a similar assessment to the Web. Reliability, the most important standard for looking critically at the Web, is discussed last.

Power and Explanatory Efficacy

The *power* of a practice is measured by its ability to help people find true answers to the questions that interest them. After the printing press increased the availability of many more books, people could use these books to increase the total amount of their knowledge. The printing press eliminated the tedious chore of copying books, giving scholars more time to produce new knowledge rather than merely duplicating the old. They could compare and cross-reference different books, rather than produce commentaries on isolated works. The sixteenth-century Danish astronomer Tycho Brahe took advantage of the printing press to detect anomalies in old records, to enlist collaborators, and to make corrections in successive additions. Scientists are concerned not only with observational truths but also with finding explanatory theories that tie together numerous observations. Placing books in the hands of scholars provided them with information that made possible assemblages of information that were united to form new theories. Darwin's realization that natural selection could be the mechanism of biological evolution was inspired by reading Malthus's work on population growth. The printing press thus contributed to the capacity of science to produce theoretical explanations by providing more scientists with more of the conceptual pieces needed to assemble new theories.

The World Wide Web is similarly powerful in helping scientists find answers to the questions that interest them. The full range of representational techniques now available on the Web can help people find answers that would otherwise be unavailable. Suppose, for example, that you want to understand binary pulsars. A new electronic astronomy journal includes a video simulation: "You will see how two stars rotate around each other: They evolve; one star sucks up matter from the other, explodes in a supernova explosion, and so on. It is a very beautiful way to illustrate a theoretical model" (Taubes 1996). Similarly, if you are curious about the operation of the new kind of bacteria that have recently been found to be a major cause of stomach ulcers, you can view an animation of *Helicobacter pylori* (available at http://www.helico.com/).

Web sites can use hypertext organization to enhance researchers' ability to find answers. The Tree of Life, for example, provides information on many species of animals and plants, organized so that browsers can easily traverse the tree up from a species to a genus or down from a genus to a species (available at http://phylogeny.arizona.edu/tree/phylogeny.html). Following hypertext links can serendipitously lead to new sources of information previously unknown to the user. The immense and rapidly increasing size of the Web, however, can limit its power. People can get so lost in following one link after another that they become "Web potatoes"—so caught up in chasing the next bit of information that they lose track of the questions they wanted to answer.

Unlike printed materials, digital databases can be searched quickly and thoroughly. The entire Web can be searched for information using numerous search engines as such Yahoo! and AltaVista, which have become available in the past few years. Scientists can use such search engines to find sites that are presenting information relevant to their own work. For researchers on such projects as the Human Genome Project, huge databases containing genetic information can yield useful answers because they are accompanied by search engines that enable users to find answers to their questions about particular genes and diseases. It is not just that search engines enable people to find information more quickly—in large scientific databases, they enable people to find answers that they would otherwise not find at all.

E-mail and news groups also are potential sources of power when they are used to solicit answers to interesting questions. Many Internet users subscribe to list servers that enable them to send e-mail automatically to people with similar interests. For example, I subscribe to a list on the psychology of science to which I can send queries or announcements. Many news groups are available for people to participate in discussions that interest them. Unmoderated news groups, to which anyone can send any message, often fill up with junk, but there are science news groups that have a moderator who screens out worthless postings, leaving entries that are likely to be relevant to researcher's work. (Compare the difference between moderated news groups such as sci.physics.research and unmoderated, junk-laden groups such as sci.physics.) Web conferences provide an even more immediate way researchers can communicate with each other to generate answers to questions of common interest.

Software easily available on the Web becomes another source of power when scientists use these programs to generate answers to statistical or other questions that would be otherwise unanswerable. Software availability will rapidly increase when more Java applications become available. The advantage of Java programs is that they run on any computer with a Web browser, eliminating the need for separate programs for Unix computers, PCs, Macintoshes, and so on.

Electronic preprint archives of the sort now available for physicists also increase scientists' ability to find answers to interesting questions. The physics archive can be searched by author and title, enabling scientists to find papers related to their questions. A similar archive is now being established for cognitive science (available at http://cogprints.soton.ac.uk/). Even without a special archive, scientists can use the general search engines on the Web to find answers to questions on an astonishing array of topics, from aardvarks to medicine to zoos. Increasing numbers of scientific journals are available on line, with searchable tables of contents and links from article to article that make it very easy to hunt down sources of information.

The Internet can also encourage the development of new theoretical ideas, as in the following example reported by Herb Brody (available at http://web.mit.edu/techreview/www/articles/oct96/brody.html; see also Brody 1996):

> Physicist Andrew Strominger . . . wrote a paper that suggested a radical departure from Einstein's conception of space-time as a smooth and continuous surface. Strominger e-mailed a question about the subject to Brian Green, who pursues similar research at Cornell. Green started to answer Strominger's question, then read the article, which Strominger had just posted on the Internet. The two scientists entered into a brief interchange of e-mail, joined by David Morrison of Duke University, and three days later all three had cowritten and posted a second paper that further refined their theory showing that tiny black holes can be transformed mathematically into infinitesimal vibrating loops of energy, called superstrings.

There are undoubtedly numerous other examples of new theoretical contributions arising from Internet-based collaborations.

Fecundity

The *fecundity* of a practice is its ability to lead to large numbers of true beliefs for *many* practitioners. This standard says that a practice should lead to truths for many people, as the printing press clearly did by making books available to far more people than previously had access to them. The number of books produced jumped to more than thirty-thousand editions by the year 1500. Astronomers, anatomists and other investigators could publish their observations for use by others. Books no longer needed to be kept locked in chests or chained in libraries.

The Internet and the World Wide Web satisfy the standard of fecundity to the extent that they provide answers for many people. Some critics have seen these technologies as providing information for the technological elite but generating yet another barrier to economic and social opportunity for residents of underdeveloped countries and the underprivileged in developed countries. But just as the printing press made books available to many who previously lacked access to university collections, so the World Wide Web makes information available to those who previously lacked access to good libraries. Physicists in underdeveloped countries whose libraries cannot afford increasingly expensive scientific journals can have the same instant access to papers that their peers in developed countries enjoy. Computers and Internet connections are not free, but they are much cheaper than travel to main libraries or purchasing or copying numerous books and journals (see under *Efficiency*). When Java applications become more widely available, special hardware or software will not be required to run them, so many people will be able to use them to help answer their questions. News groups and e-mail lists reach many people simultaneously and can therefore contribute to the ability of many people to find answers to their questions. Web conferences and on-line forums have the potential to increase the knowledge of many people.

The potential fecundity of the World Wide Web is illustrated by the Cancer Genome Anatomy Project of the National Cancer Institute (available at http:// inhouse.ncbi.nlm.nih.gov/ncicgap/). This interdisciplinary project aims to establish the information and technological tools needed to decipher the molecular anatomy of cancer cells. Because cancer is now known to be a molecular-genetic disease (see chapter 2), detailed understanding of the genes involved in cancerous cells may well lead to effective new treatments. The National Cancer Institute (NCI) is using the Web as its main means of disseminating information about genes that affect different kinds of tumors:

> The NCI will make all Tumor Gene Index Project resources (database, libraries and sequences) immediately available to the cancer community for uses such as monitoring of gene expression in tumors. The intent is that the Tumor Gene Index

will be a comprehensive resource to the cancer research community, providing an unprecedented link between the molecular anatomy and pathology of cancer. The focal point for communication with the community will be the Cancer Genome Anatomy Project Web Page. Through this resource cancer researchers will be able to access information relating to all aspects of the Cancer Genome Anatomy Project ranging from a broad overview of the program, to information about resources produced by the project, to opportunities to participate in the project. Most importantly, the web page will provide specific information with respect to how the community can access DNA sequences, cDNA libraries, and arrayed clones. A unique feature of the web page will be a "hot technology" section describing the latest developments of the Tumor Gene Index in informatics, library production, microdissection or rapid array hybridization. (available at: http://inhouse.ncbi. nlm.nih.gov/ncicgap/intro.html)

All the Cancer Genome Anatomy Project information is available to anyone with a Web browser, and the project can therefore increase the knowledge of many researchers and medical practitioners.

Speed

The *speed* of a practice is how quickly it leads to true answers. People aim to acquire knowledge quickly as well as reliably; the printing press, for example, contributed enormously to the speed with which knowledge could be disseminated. No longer did scholars need to travel to distant libraries to consult rare copies of books, since printed books were produced in sufficient numbers that they could be held in numerous places. Scholars could even have their own copies of books, enabling them to increase their knowledge without the time needed to consult libraries. Printed tables of logarithmic functions spared astronomers much calculating time. Production of printed books increased the size of libraries and encouraged the use of full alphabetical order and indexes, leading to speedier searches for information.

The Internet and the World Wide Web have enormous advantages over other resources for information with respect to the speed of producing answers. Electronic mail can transfer information around the world in seconds or minutes, in contrast to the days or weeks required for communication by traditional mail. When scientific information is posted on a Web site such as OMIM or sent to a preprint archive, it becomes available instantly, in contrast to the months or even years that publication in books and journals can take. The entire World Wide Web and many Web databases have search engines that provide information with a speed that was unimaginable a decade ago. New applications such as Java offer the potential for speedy use of new software.

Of course, as everyone who has used the Web knows, the speed of Internet use is heavily affected by the extent of usage at a particular moment. Information that might be almost instantaneously available at 6 A.M. may be painfully slow to load later, when many more people are accessing the Internet. The World Wide Web has been called the World Wide Wait. Information seekers may waste time chasing one link after another when a trip to the library would more quickly tell them what they want to know. The many entertaining sites on the Web may distract people from looking for the information they need and slow down their work rather than speed it up. But used intelligently, the World Wide Web can be the most rapid source of information ever available.

Efficiency

The *efficiency* of a practice is how well it limits the cost of obtaining true answers. Copying books by hand consumed huge amounts of labor, whereas printing made possible the distribution of books at a fraction of the cost.

A friend once suggested that WWW stands for "Wicked Waste of We-sources." Using the Internet is indeed costly because of the computers and information storage required, but it nevertheless fares well on the standard of efficiency. E-mail, news groups, and electronic archives are much cheaper than sending paper mail. It is much less costly for CERN's international research groups to communicate electronically and access information from a common Web server than to try to meet frequently and exchange data using physical tapes. Papers can now be stored electronically for less than a thousandth of a cent per page, far cheaper than paper storage and reproduction. Expensive computer and network connections are not efficient for an organization whose members are using them to download recipes, play multiple-user games, and learn more about their favorite television shows. But the increasing amount of valuable information on the Web, including scientific information, makes it a highly efficient source of true answers if used intelligently.

The power, fecundity, speed, and efficiency of the Internet are impressive, but they raise problems about the quality of information that are even more severe than those that arose with the advent of print and television. Anyone with a Web site can post virtually anything, and a random look at what Joe Hacker has to say about the origin of the universe may be worse than useless. Web pages and postings to unmoderated news groups (e.g., the claim on alt.conspiracy that flight TWA 800 was shot down by the U.S. Navy) undergo no screening and evaluation, whereas even a profit-driven book or magazine publisher or cable television provider has to apply some standards of taste and credibility. Libraries and other purchasers apply standards when they decide what is worth buying and making available to readers. In contrast, the lack of screening on the Web is accompanied by an unprecedented degree of access by anyone who has a connection to the Internet. Similarly, some newsgroups and e-mail list servers are overwhelmed by contributions from people who type faster than they think. Compared with print and television, the Internet provides less scrutiny and more access, so the problem of distinguishing knowledge and nonsense is even more acute.

Reliability and Pragmatic Efficacy

The *reliability* of a practice is measured by the ratio of truths to the total number of beliefs fostered by the practice, and the printing press increased reliability in several ways. The previous method of producing books by hand copying inevitably introduced mistakes, whereas a press could produce many copies of a book without introducing any new errors. Moreover, the wide availability of printed books encouraged readers to consider the extent to which the contents of the book were accurate reflections of nature, rather than taking the contents of the books as sacrosanct. When errors crept into printed books, errata could be published and distributed to scattered readers. Illustrations could be duplicated exactly, instead of depending on the varying ability of each copier to reproduce drawings exactly. Before printing, maps were frequently unreliable, because copying by hand introduced distortions and inaccuracies. The printing press greatly increased the reliability of scientific communication.

Of course, the printing press was and is a mixed blessing. From the beginning, it was used to promulgate nonsense as well as knowledge. Shoddy books on worthless topics could sap the time and energy of thinkers and fill their minds with error. Books on astrology were as likely to attract the printer looking for a profitable product as books on empirical astronomy; in fact, horoscopes were published shortly after Gutenberg's bible, well before the publication of astronomical observations. Nevertheless, the overall contribution of the printing press to the production and availability of scientific knowledge is clear, according to the standards of reliability, power, fecundity, speed, and efficiency.

How do the Web and other Internet technologies improve the reliability of the research of scientists like Marie Darwin? Various technologies can help her avoid erroneous beliefs. By e-mailing notes and drafts of papers to her students and collaborators, she can get immediate feedback that can lead her to correct misconceptions before they become entrenched in her thinking. Similarly, sending her preprints to an electronic archive gives other researchers a chance to examine her work and suggest improvements. Conferencing over the Web provides another way in which the reliability of Marie's work can benefit from the critical response of her collaborators. Science, like knowledge in general, is an inherently social enterprise in which achieving truth and avoiding error gains enormously from feedback that Internet technologies can help provide.

Seeking information generally on the World Wide Web is not always a reliable practice. But in the hands of scientists and other careful users, posting information on the Web has several features that can increase reliability. Unlike books and journals, which are sent out into the world permanently, information on the Web can be easily updated and corrected. Whereas printed information needs to wait for further publications or new editions to correct errors, changes to a Web site can be made quickly to prevent propagation of erroneous information. Experimental databases such as those used at CERN and in the Human Genome Project can undergo continuous expansion and correction. Preprint archives are a potential source of misinformation, since the papers sent to them do not undergo the careful reviewing process that precedes journal publication. This problem may turn out to be more acute for psychology than for physics, whose journals have lower rejection rates than psychology journals—a physics paper is probably going to end up published anyway. But the potential for introduction of errors is to some extent compensated for by the ease with which new preprints and e-mailing among researchers can help correct earlier mistakes.

Many scientific fields, such as chemistry, involve objects whose three-dimensional and dynamic character are inadequately captured by verbal and two-dimensional representations. More reliable information may sometimes be provided by special Web tools such as virtual reality browsers that provide much richer three-dimensional information. Videos and animations can provide more realistic depictions of the motions of a system under investigation. Like any picture, virtual reality displays and animations can provide erroneous impressions, but they have the potential to provide more accurate representations of the inherently three-dimensional and dynamic aspects of the world that they describe. These examples show that the World Wide Web can both increase and diminish reliability. But even more than readers of printed sources, Web users need intellectual tools for discriminating between reliable and unreliable sources of information.

For medical information, the World Wide Web has a number of superb sources of information that can contribute to the pragmatic efficacy of the practices of physicians and patients. These include:

- Medscape (http://www.medscape.com/), which provides summary articles and access to Medline, the online index of publications in medical journals
- The Doctor's Guide to the Internet (http://www.pslgroup.com/docguide.htm), which includes numerous links to other medical sites
- CancerNet (http://www.icic.nci.nih.gov/), which provides comprehensive information from the U.S. National Cancer Institute

These sites provide access to reliable information on numerous diseases. NIH Consensus Statements produced by the conferences discussed in the last chapter are also available (http://odp.od.nih.gov/consensus/). There are hundreds of additional sites with valuable medical information, such as Barry Marshall's site on *H. pylori* (available at http://www.helico.com/). At the other extreme, there are countless sources of medical nonsense on the Web, touting dubious medical treatments such as homeopathy, which is mentioned in more than ten thousand Web documents.

CONCLUSION

This chapter was inspired by my realization of how useful the World Wide Web was becoming for my own research: See chapters 5, 6, and 12 for references to some of the sites that have helped my study of the ulcers case. Previously, I found the Internet valuable mostly for e-mail. The collaboration with Keith Holyoak described in chapter 12 was primarily accomplished by e-mail; we wrote our book *Mental Leaps* with only one face-to-face meeting and only a handful of phone conversations, sending chapter drafts back and forth electronically.

Table 13.1 summarizes how various Internet technologies can contribute to scientific research. There is great variation in the extent to which these technologies are now being used. Every scientific field now has available to it e-mail, news groups, and World Wide Web sites, but only physics has an extensive preprint archive. Within different fields, there is also great variability in the extent to which different scientists use technologies such as Web-based databases. For the Human Genome Project and particle physics at CERN, such databases have become essential, but other scientific projects that are less collaborative can handle their data locally in more traditional ways. Visualization using graphically oriented browsers is becoming important for fields such as biomedicine but may have little impact on other fields. Some of the technologies I have mentioned, such as Java applications, virtual reality browsers, and Web conferencing are new and have so far received little use, although all have promising futures.

In describing these various ways in which Internet technologies such as the World Wide Web can contribute to scientific knowledge, I have provided a positive model of how the technologies can be used to foster the development of knowledge in anyone, including nonscientists such as students. At the other extreme, there is the real and frightening prospect of students and other people wasting electronic resources to fill their heads with nonsense gleaned from the many worthless sites on the Web. Internet epistemology includes the highly critical task of examining and evaluating the large quantities of pseudoscience that the Web is being used to promulgate. My purpose in this chapter has been more positive; to describe the Internet at its best in aiding the development of scientific knowledge.

TABLE 13.1
Summary of the Contributions of Internet Technologies to Scientific Research

	Reliability	*Power*	*Speed*	*Fecundity*	*Efficiency*
E-mail, news groups	Feedback for corrections	Many answers available	Faster than paper mail	Multiple recipients	Cheaper than paper mail
Hypertext (the Web)	Easily revised	Follow links, use search engines	Instant publishing; no wait for access, searching	Widely available, distance irrelevant	Storage cheap
Animation, video, VRML (virtual reality modeling language)	More accurate depiction of structures and motion	Lots of visual information not otherwise available			
Java	Software not under local control	Instant provision of software to conduct examination, searches	No wait for software	Use by everyone, regardless of kind of computer	No need to buy software or to spend time downloading it
Databases	Updatable, verifiable	Huge amount of information available	Fast searchers, instant availability	Accessible to many	Storage cheap
Preprint archives	Potentially rapid feedback	Access latest research results	Instant access	Journal access unnecessary	Total cost much lower than for print
Conferencing	Immediate corrections	Combine new ideas	No need to meet	Everyone involved	Cheaper than meeting

SUMMARY

In recent years, Internet technologies such as electronic mail and the World Wide Web have dramatically affected scientific communication and collaboration. Many researchers use these technologies in their day-to-day research, and these resources are essential to organizations such as the Human Genome Project and CERN. There are thousands of science-related sites on the World Wide Web, including an archive of physics papers that has become one of the main methods by which physicists communicate the results of their research. The Web and other technologies enable many researchers to generate answers to questions with speed and efficiency. Although the reliability of information on the Web is suspect because of the numerous sites of low quality, careful use of the Web and the Internet in general can help increase and spread knowledge in science and medicine.

Part Five

CONCLUSION

CHAPTER 14

Science as a Complex System

I SUGGESTED in chapter 1 that the traditional view of science as logic and the postmodern view of science as power are both inadequate for understanding how science develops. Their inadequacy was evident in chapters 3 to 6, which described the connected psychological, social, and physical processes that produced the discovery and acceptance of the bacterial theory of ulcers, when Barry Marshall and Robin Warren collaborated to produce observations and experiments that helped change their minds and the minds of others. Chapters 7 to 10 explored cognitive processes involved in causal reasoning and conceptual change, and chapters 11 to 13 provided further discussion of social processes. It should be obvious by now that science is a complex psychological, social, and physical system. The complexity of the system derives from both (1) the heterogeneity of its parts, which range from mental representations to social institutions to instruments to organisms, and (2) the intricacy of the organization and interactions of these parts.

Such complexity hinders the task of describing more generally how the system works. The Integrated Cognitive-Social Explanation Schema in chapter 1 needs to be fleshed out to characterize more fully how psychological and social processes interact, and it needs to be supplemented to reflect how these processes are affected by scientists' physical interactions with the world. As I argued in chapter 5, bacteria are neither mental nor social creations; they evolved hundreds of millions of years before people and their societies came on the scene. The story of the rise of the bacterial theory of ulcers has to include the role of physical entities such as *Helicobacter pylori*, stomachs, and the instruments used to observe them. Of course, the use of instruments, observation, and experimentation is not detached from the mental and social aspects of science, but it is not reducible to them either. A more adequate depiction of the influences on the development of scientific knowledge is shown in Figure 14.1. If we want to understand the development of scientific knowledge, we need to understand not only the effects of mind, society, and nature on the growth of science but also the mutual influences among the three kinds of factors. Figure 14.1, however, is more a logo than a theory. To provide some content to the arrows requires more than detailed examination of particular cases in the history of science, such as the bacterial theory of ulcers. It also requires developing new models of science as a complex system that characterize the arrows more generally.

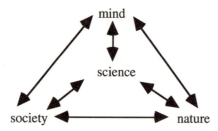

Figure 14.1. Science as a complex system. Arrows indicate mutual causal influences.

The study of science, like science itself, often resorts to metaphors and analogies to suggest new models. The first task of this concluding chapter is to examine several metaphors and analogies that have been proposed to make sense of the complexities of scientific practice. The next section assesses the advantages and disadvantages of characterizing science as a motley, a mangle, an ecology, an actor network, and a trading zone. I then present what I think is a superior analogy for understanding science as a complex system, using the idea of distributed computation to further the integration of different ways of understanding science. The psychological and social dimensions of science can be connected by viewing scientific research as akin to distributed artificial intelligence (DAI), with the development of ideas in science and medicine construed as parts of a complex computational system. DAI is a relatively new branch of the field of artificial intelligence that concerns how problems can be solved by networks of intelligent computers that communicate with each other. Although I assume the cognitivist view that individual scientists are information processors, I argue that the view of a scientific community as a network of information processors is not reductionist and does not eliminate or subordinate the role of sociologists or social historians in understanding science. I conclude with a discussion of the contentious issues of rationality and realism, completing my argument that attention to the psychological and social complexities of scientific practice does not undermine the validity of scientific knowledge.

METAPHORS AND ANALOGIES IN SCIENCE STUDIES

From the ancient discovery that sound behaves like water waves to Darwin's use of the analogy between natural and artificial selection, metaphors and analogies have made great contributions to the growth of scientific knowledge (Holyoak and Thagard 1995 [chapter 8]). It is not surprising, then, that philosophers, historians, psychologists, sociologists, and others striving to understand the complexities of science have resorted to a wide range of metaphors and analogies. These are valuable when they highlight the nature and interactions of important factors in the development of science, but they can also limit understanding when they impede recognition of other contributors. All the conceptualizations discussed in this section are superior to monolithic views of science as *just* logic or power or psychology or sociology, but they vary in the extent to which they point to richer views.

Motleys and Mangles

Wittgenstein (1956, p. 88) said that he wanted to give an account of the "motley of mathematics," and Hacking (1992, p. 29) wrote of the "motley of the sciences" before commenting on general characteristics of the laboratory sciences. The motley metaphor suggests that science is composed of diverse, incongruous strands and that simple and accurate generalizations about it are rare. This metaphor is useful in directing us to look for the complexities of science, but it provides no guidance in how to understand those complexities.

The diversity of science is also suggested by the strange title of Pickering's book(1995), *The Mangle of Practice*. Pickering (1992) announced a shift from understanding science as knowledge to understanding it as practice, and for his book he took the mangle metaphor from an old-fashioned device used to squeeze the water out of clothes being washed. He employed the metaphor to highlight the unpredictable material and social transformations that occur in science. Emphasis on the varied activities of scientists is useful when it focuses attention on the diverse ways in which scientists interact with the world and develop knowledge of it. Like most sociologists, however, Pickering has little to say about the cognitive processes that scientists use to learn about the world.

For most of the twentieth century, both philosophy and sociology have been psychophobic, steering away from discussions of the operations of the mind. For philosophers in the logical tradition, the fear has been that attention to psychological matters would undermine objectivity and rationality. For sociologists, the fear has been that admission of psychological explanations would reductively render sociological explanations superfluous. Both these fears are groundless, but understanding of the relations between the psychological and the sociological requires rich metaphors that do not mangle science by ignoring the minds of scientists and the world in which they work.

Ecologies

Ecology is the branch of science that deals with the interrelationships of organisms and their environment. Because it is concerned not only with individual organisms but with groups of organisms, such as members of a species, and because it considers organisms in interaction with the world in which they live, ecology is an attractive potential source of analogies for science studies. Hence, it is not surprising that Campbell (1988) and Hull (1989) espouse evolutionary models of science, that Kitcher (1993) borrows mathematical tools from population biology to analyze the division of cognitive labor, and that Fujimura (1996) discusses the development of ideas about cancer in terms of "ecologies of action."

Ecological analogies may be suggestive about the social and environmental aspects of science, but they tend to distract attention from psychological processes that operate in humans. There is evidence that humans are the only organisms capable of sophisticated analogies (Holyoak and Thagard 1995 [chapter 3]), and the other kinds of high-level cognition used by scientists in the formation and evaluation of hypotheses may also be specific to our species. Hence, ecological and evolutionary approaches that ignore the cognitive capacities of humans are of limited use in understanding the complexities of psychosocial relations in science.

Actor Networks

Callon (1986) and Latour (1987) have propounded a potentially richer metaphor of science as a network of actors and have applied it to a variety of cases involving the development of science and technology. The network metaphor serves well to highlight social aspects of science, such as the way scientists enlist each other's help in spreading their views, but Callon and Latour have an odd way of bringing the world into their networks. Denying any division between the social and the natural, they treat objects in the world as actors, or, as they say, *actants*. Scientists are actants in the scientific network, but so are the things and organisms they study. They avoid the exaggerations of the claim that science is merely a social construction, but they do so at the cost of giving bacteria and other nonhuman actants the same cognitive status as human scientists. Without recognition that scientists differ from bacteria in having minds that they use to think about the world, the actor-network metaphor is woefully limited in its ability to explain the complexities of science.

Trading Zones

In his rich and detailed discussion of the practices of twentieth-century physics, Galison (1997) provides a novel and fertile analogy for understanding the diverse groups of experimenters and theoreticians, describing their interactions in terms of the trading zones described by anthropologists:

> Subcultures trade. Anthropologists have extensively studied how different groups, with radically different ways of dividing up the world and symbolically

organizing its parts, can not only exchange goods but also depend essentially on those trades. Within a certain cultural arena—what I call in chapter 9 the "trading zone"—two dissimilar groups can find common ground. They can exchange fish for baskets, enforcing subtle equations of correspondence between quantity, quality, and type, and yet utterly disagree on the broader (global) significance of the items exchanged. Similarly, between the scientific subcultures of theory and experiment, or even between different traditions of instrument making or different subcultures of theorizing, there can be exchanges (coordinations), worked out in exquisite local detail, without global agreement. (Galison 1997, p. 46)

He uses this analogy to construct an insightful analysis of the interactions of theory and experimentation that appreciates their importance to the development of physics while also taking seriously the material constraints provided by the world. It would be natural to reframe my account of the development of the bacterial theory of ulcers in terms of the trading zones among gastroenterologists, microbiologists, and other researchers.

Like most historians of science, however, Galison says little about the psychological processes used by scientists in their interactions. His trading zone metaphor clearly does not exclude such processes: There is a whole field of cognitive anthropology that investigates the psychological underpinnings of cultural differences (D'Andrade 1995). Just as anthropologists can map the cognitive structures of the different cultures interacting in a trading zone, so the psychology of science can consider the cognitive structures of the different groups of scientists whose collaboration is essential for progress in modern science. The trading zone metaphor has room for minds as well as society and the world. But, like the rest of the metaphors for the diversity and complexity of science considered in this section, it does little to generate a model of social-psychological interactions.

DISTRIBUTED COMPUTATION

In modern cognitive science, the dominant analogy is between the mind and the computer, exploiting parallels between the representations and operations of the mind and the structures and algorithms of computer programs (Thagard 1996, chapters 1–7). For a full understanding of science, the cognitive framework needs to be expanded to fit into a broader explanatory scheme that encompasses the social. According to cognitivism, thinking is computation. Hence, individual scientists can be viewed as computers that communicate with each other through various means. Cognitivism does not, of course, assume that people are just like any of the computers we currently have. Human intelligence still far outstrips computer intelligence in most respects, and it is reasonable to expect that radically different hardware and software from what is currently available will be necessary before computers reach human levels of intelligence. During the 1990s, much of the most interesting research in cognitive science has used models inspired in part by the sort of parallel computation among highly connected units that occurs in the brain. I view these connectionist approaches as cognitivist, even though they assume a very different view of computation than some approaches that are traditional to artificial intelligence. If, as is argued by various critics of artificial intelligence and cognitive science, computational ideas miss fundamental aspects of human intelligence, then cognitivism will ultimately fail as an approach to the psychology of thinking. But cognitivism has greatly enhanced our understanding of numerous kinds of thinking, and it needs to be supplemented with ideas about social and dynamic systems rather than replaced (Thagard 1996 [chapters 10–11]).

The proliferation of networks of computers has spawned a new subfield of artificial intelligence concerned with how problems can be solved cooperatively by means of interacting computers. In a simple computer network, each computer is a node, and communication takes place between computers through rapid transmission of information digitally encoded. DAI investigates how a network of computers, each possessing some degree of intelligence, can collectively have accomplishments that no individual computer could easily have on its own (Bond and Gasser 1988; Durfee et al. 1989; Gasser 1991; Hewitt 1991; O'Hare and Jennings 1996).

Even among digital computers, communication is restricted because of bandwidth limitations or the high computational cost of sending information. Computer networks are becoming increasingly complex; for example, the Andrew network at Carnegie Mellon University includes thousands of nodes distributed over fifty-five buildings. The computers communicate with each other by means of more than one hundred subnetworks, including Ethernet and Apple Talk connections. Many artificial intelligence applications are inherently distributed, for example, controling a set of intelligent robots that work together or bring together a number of expert systems with complementary areas of expertise. Distributed computing differs from parallel computing in that the latter typically involves simple nodes of similar kinds communicating with each other in straightforward ways. In connectionist systems, for example, each neuron-like node is an uncomplicated device that updates its activation based on the activation of the nodes to which it is linked and also the weights on those links (Rumelhart and McClelland 1986). Intelligence is an emergent property of the operation of numerous interacting nodes, not of each individual node. In contrast, in distributed artificial intelligence it is assumed that each node has much greater computational power than the simple units in connectionist systems, including the capacity to communicate in more complicated ways with other nodes. DAI nodes are usually called *agents* and are endowed with much greater cognitive capacity than the "actants" of Callon and Latour.

Remarkably, researchers in DAI have turned to sociology for ideas about how to describe the organization and functioning of computer networks. One early paper developed ideas about distributed computing by using scientific communities as a metaphor (Kornfeld and Hewitt 1981). More recent papers by Hewitt (1991) and Gasser (1991) include respectful references to such sociologists as Garfinkel, Gerson, and Latour. The use of sociological concepts by researchers in DAI is consistent with the kind of unified model of science that I envision, since my intention is not to reduce the sociology of science to distributed computation but to provide a unifying framework that ties together sociological insights with cognitive ones. But whereas Kornfeld and Hewitt used scientific communities as an analog to help understand parallel and distributed computing, I work the analogy in the opposite direction and construct a more elaborate model of scientific communities. The bidirectional application of the analogy between societies and computer networks is similar to the bidirectional use of the analogy between minds and computers, which has been exploited in different ways at different times depending on the current state of knowledge in the two domains. Early ideas about computers were inspired in part by early models of neurons, and important ideas in artificial intelligence were inspired by studies of human problem solving. On the other hand, computational ideas have proved invaluable in developing and specifying models of human cognition. During the 1980s, the direction of the analogy was reversed again, as connectionists found computational inspiration in brain-like operations. Bidirectional analogies enable two different fields to progress together by exploiting advances in one field to bring the other forward in a process of mutual bootstrapping.

To make plausible a view of science as distributed computing, we need to identify the main nodes and communication channels that occur in scientific communities. To avoid a purely abstract characterization, I sketch a single example concerning the field of experimental cognitive psychology. A similar account could easily be given of many other fields, including medical research; my choice is not intended to give my account any kind of cognitive bias but merely reflects my familiarity with the field.

Let us start with individual scientists, treating each as a node in a communication network. Communication between scientists is not so easy as the digital communication that can take place between conventional computers, as we cannot simply transmit information from the brain of one scientist to another. Information is transmitted, however, through personal contact between scientists or more indirectly through journals and other publications. As described in chapter 13, scholarly communication is becoming increasingly electronic. Communication requires extensive coding and decoding, as scientists attempt to put what they know into words or pictures that other scientists must attempt to understand. Obviously, each scientist must be viewed as a very complex computational system, capable of not only solving problems but also producing and understanding speech, diagrams, and written text. Each scientist communicates directly with only a relatively small number of other scientists, although publication greatly increases the possible lines of communication.

Starting with scientists as nodes, we can try to draw graphs that identify the communication links between them. Nodes will form clusters, since there will be subgroups of scientists that are more tightly interconnected than the group as a whole. Among cognitive psychologists, for example, there are at least the four following kinds of subgroups:

1. *Collaborators.* Scientists at the same or different institution who are working on common projects communicate frequently (see chapter 11).

2. *Students and teachers.* Communication links exist between scientists and scientists in training. If, as in cognitive psychology and many other fields, the students function as collaborators on research projects, the links are particularly tight. Research methods and skills are communicated along with more easily described verbal information.

3. *Colleagues.* Scientist working in the same university department may see each other regularly and exchange ideas.

4. *Acquaintances.* Scientists who regularly attend the same conferences and workshops get to know each other and may exchange information irregularly.

One powerful source of ongoing communication links involves students who were previously students together. A high proportion of the most influential current practitioners in cognitive psychology received their graduate training at a small number of universities, such as Stanford, Michigan, and Harvard. More intermittent direct communication can occur between scientists who attend conferences or visit campuses to give colloquia.

Indirect communication links between individual scientists can exist by virtue of publications. Although there are numerous psychology journals, some are far more influential than others. Cognitive psychologists know that a paper is far more likely to be read if it appears in *Psychological Review* or *Cognitive Psychology* than if it appears in a more obscure location. Figure 14.2 depicts a small part of a processing network in a scientific community. The scientists at the top form a cluster, perhaps because they are colleagues at the same institution. They have direct links to each other, but only one has a direct link with a member of another cluster. By publishing in and reading in the journal, however, indirect communication is established between other scientists. Given the years it can take to get a paper written, published, and read, this is a much slower form of communication than direct exchange, but its importance is undeniable.

Somewhat faster exchange takes place through communication by presentation at conferences. For experimental cognitive psychologists, the most impor-

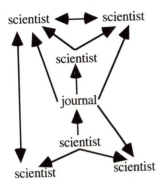

Figure 14.2. Communication in a small part of a scientific community, through personal contact or by publishing in and reading journals.

tant meeting is the annual conference of the Psychonomics Society, but conferences of the Cognitive Science Society, the American Psychological Society, and ad hoc groups also provide occasions for the dissemination of research results and personal interactions. As described in chapter 13, Internet technologies provide numerous ways of maintaining contacts and increasing the rapid flow of information. The sort of network I am describing is much richer than that of Latour (1987), who talks of networks of scientists and their inscriptions without allowing that each node is a highly complex processing system.

My discussion is consistent with the view that scientific communities constitute "invisible colleges" (Crane 1972), but it integrates considerations of social organization with the obvious fact that the individual scientists are cognitive beings. In short, scientific communities are societies of minds. Other vehicles for indirect communication exist. Book chapters, especially those that provide authoritative reviews of work in particular fields, can be important. Monographs and textbooks can also become widely read and important for communicating with a broad group of scientists. To carry out research that involves the paying of subjects, computer equipment, and other expenses, scientists need to obtain grants. They must therefore send proposals to funding agencies such as the National Science Foundation; these agencies then send the proposals to other scientists for review, and the other scientists communicate their opinion back to the agency, which makes a decision. Because over time new scientists enter each field and new lines of communication arise between established scientists, the system of computational nodes and links is constantly evolving.

Not all communication is best described as the sharing of information. In distributed artificial intelligence, it is not unusual for computers to be in conflict with each other, and DAI researchers have emphasized the importance of how computers can negotiate with each other to overcome conflicts. Negotiation among members of scientific communities includes discussions between journal editors and authors concerning whether articles will be published. Leading psychology journals rarely accept manuscripts as submitted, and more than one round of reviewing is common. An author is often asked to revise and resubmit a manuscript and to revise it further if it is accepted conditionally. Negotiations also take place in decisions concerning funding. As part of a theory of adversarial problem solving, Thagard (1992a) sketched some of the cognitive mechanisms that are relevant to negotiation, including developing a model of an opponent. Latour (1987) has described sociological aspects of the adversarial side of science: Scientists attempt to mobilize allies and resources to increase their strength relative to opposing groups. It would be a mistake, however, to emphasize the competitive nature of science to the neglect of the cooperative side. Chapter 11 described the enormous extent to which science is based on trust, not just within particular research groups but across whole fields. No researcher can check all experimental and theoretical conclusions alone, so there is enormous dependency both within and across groups.

Using the framework so far developed, we could in principle draw a graph that specifies the connections among all members of a field, such as cognitive psychology or gastroenterology. Of course, each field does not compose a closed system, and there would have to be links to scientists and journals in allied areas. For example, many cognitive psychologists pay attention to work in related areas of psychology such as social and developmental psychology, and a smaller number read in or communicate with practitioners of other disciplines, such as artificial intelligence and philosophy of mind. In sum, my proposal is that we view a scientific community as a system for distributed computation.

OBJECTIONS AND LIMITATIONS OF SCIENCE AS DISTRIBUTED COMPUTATION

The most obvious objection to using distributed computation as a social model of science is that it presupposes the use of computation as a model of individual psychology. Whether intelligence should be understood computationally and whether there is any hope for the development of artificial intelligence have been challenged by critics such as Collins (1990) and Dreyfus (1992). Such criticisms have often been useful for pointing out gaps and oversimplifications in computational approaches to cognition, but artificial intelligence and the computational modeling of human cognition are highly dynamic fields. Collins's critique is largely based on an examination of rule-based expert systems, a 1970s technology that gained widespread industrial use in the 1980s. In the 1980s and 1990s, there have been various developments that show promise of helping artificial intelligence overcome the inflexibility and poor performance that has characterized many past systems.

I have already alluded to one development, distributed artificial intelligence, which is helping overcome artificial intelligence's traditional neglect of social questions. Artificial intelligence has also tended to neglect questions of embodiment of intelligent systems and real-world interactions, but there has been increasing research on incorporating artificial intelligence ideas in robotic systems to produce autonomous mechanical agents (Mackworth 1993; Moravec 1988). Simple artificial intelligence programs have neglected the fact that human intelligence depends on vast amounts of commonsense knowledge, but an attempt has been made to compile a huge and well-organized database of commonsense knowledge that can provide background information for complex inferencing (Lenat and Guha 1990). In 1980, there was only scattered work on how computer programs could learn, but machine learning is now an active subfield within artificial intelligence (Langley 1996; Mitchell 1997). The 1980s also saw several approaches to developing artificial intelligence systems that differ substantially from rule-based expert systems. Connectionist systems that consist of numerous interconnected neuron-like nodes have proved powerful for a variety of tasks that are difficult for traditional artificial intelligence. Another non–rule-based approach that has received growing attention is the use of analogies with particular cases to solve problems and provide explanation (Kolodner 1993). In the area of expert systems, there have been important theoretical developments in using Bayesian belief networks for diagnostic reasoning (Pearl 1988). Other artificial intelligence researchers would point to additional developments as significant in recent work.

This is not of course to say that the problems of developing artificial intelligence and computational models of mind have been solved. Artificial intelligence's most enthusiastic cheerleaders such as Lenat and Moravec expect that the fundamental computational problems of developing computational systems will be solved within a matter of decades. My own guess is that we are still missing a number of key conceptual ingredients for understanding natural and artificial intelligence, so I would project centuries rather than decades of research. It is also possible that the problem of understanding the mind is too complex for the mind to solve, or that the computational approach is fundamentally flawed, perhaps because thought is ineluctably tacit or situated in the world. But artificial intelligence has at least the possibility of modeling tacit knowledge (through connectionist distributed representations or cases used analogically) and of situating cognition in the world (through DAI and robotics). Progress has been sufficient in the past few decades that the only reasonable collective scientific strategy is to wait and see how the ideas play themselves out.

One obvious requisite of a serious model of science as distributed computation is that each processor be highly complex and capable of performing at least a simplified version of the cognitive operations of scientists, including forming hypotheses, designing experiments, and evaluating theories. There are also cognitive processes involved in deciding when and how to communicate. When a scientist has completed a paper, for example, what determines the journal to which the paper is submitted for publication? Most likely, if the scientist is experienced and acute, that question will have already affected the writing of the paper, since journals vary in their subject matter, audience, and length of papers accepted. An astute publishing strategy requires that the scientist have a sophisticated view of the publication venues available, including their relative influence and accessibility.

After the question of the possibility of individual computational intelligence, the second most likely objection to my distributed computation model is that it is not really social, since the interactions of processors in distributed networks are so primitive compared with the interactions of humans. DAI is normally concerned with computers that are linked to each other by efficient networks that allow virtually instantaneous transmission of digitized information in standard formats. Transmission between humans even via conversations is much slower and involves far more encoding and decoding of knowledge than is required in digital transmission. In practice, however, DAI faces real problems in communication too, since two computers may use different representational schemes and inference engines. Communication may also require considerable encoding and decoding, even though all information is in electronic form. It might prove desirable, for example, to bring about collaboration between a rule-based expert system, a Bayesian network system, and a case-based reasoner, each with expertise in related domains. Such systems use very different ways of representing information, so that producing communication and cooperation among them is highly nontrivial and would require considerable processing.

Collins (1990, pp. 4–5) specifies several ways in which science is social. One is the "routine servicing of beliefs," in which a scientific group affects how an individual checks the validity of beliefs. It is easy to see how this could be modeled within DAI, for example, when one processor generates a hypothesis that is communicated to another processor that may reply by communicating additional evidence, counterevidence, or alternative hypotheses. Such communication also shows how Collins's second way in which science is social can be understood computationally: Conclusions to scientific debates are matters of social consensus, with potential equilibria being reached by the passing of messages back and forth until either all processors agree or are undergoing no further change. More problematic for my DAI model of science is Collins's other way in which science is social. He claims that the transfer of new experimental skills requires social intercourse rather than simply reading journal articles. This claim is certainly true for experimental cognitive psychology, in which students typically learn experimental methods not from articles, textbooks, or methods courses but from apprenticing with an experienced researcher. Similarly, medical skills such as endoscopy require hands-on instruction.

Collins's point does not, however, undermine the DAI perspective, for it can be interpreted as showing the need for some kinds of communication to be particularly intense. Intensity can be a matter of the amount of information transmitted—articles typically report much less than the experiment knows—and the format of information. One advantage of face-to-face human interaction is the ease of using visual representations: One person can draw something or simply point to a key piece of experimental equipment. Artificial intelligence has been slow to exploit the power of visual representations, but this is gradually changing (Chandrasekaran et al. 1995). There is no reason in principle, however, that artificial intelligence processors equipped with capacities for visual representation and interaction with the world could not communicate skills in the complex ways that Collins describes. Whether artificial intelligence will accomplish such communication will depend on the success of the whole research program and cannot be decided in advance.

A DAI model of science is also compatible with the view of Longino (1990) that scientific knowledge is inherently social. She advocates an antireductionist social view of science on the grounds that scientific knowledge is constructed through interactions among individuals and that individual scientists' knowledge is made possible by their social and cultural contexts. Although DAI is more easily applicable to modeling interactions within scientific communities rather than entire societies, it is rich enough to allow the values that Longino identifies as ineliminable parts of science. Values can be represented by the varying goals possessed by agents in DAI systems.

All analogies have limitations, and it must be recognized that DAI is presently only a weak approximation to the complexities of scientific practice. Existing artificial intelligence system programs do not even come close to the intellectual capabilities of individual scientists, and current DAI models that capture various kinds of collective problem solving have not been used to model scientific communities. (An exception is a project on modeling scientific group decision making that Toby Donaldson and I have under way.) The most serious limitation is that although DAI may suggest ways of integrating the psychological and the sociological, it might seem to neglect the world, since most DAI systems run on computers that have no interactions with their environments. However, there is a rapidly merging branch of DAI called *collective robotics*, which investigates how robots can work together in physical interaction with the world to solve problems such as playing soccer (available at http://diwww.epfl.ch/lami/collective/Sommaire_bibliotheque.html). The study of collective robotics is a long way from having communities of robots performing experiments and explaining their results, but it serves to provide a concrete instantiation of the possibility of computational intelligences interacting with each other and the world.

My discussion of how the social aspects of science can be interpreted within the framework of distributed computation should be viewed as taking those aspects seriously rather than as explaining them away. To make this clearer, I now show why it would be mistaken to view a DAI approach as demeaning the social by espousing reductionism or methodological individualism.

REDUCTION

As indicated in chapter 1, the question of the relation between philosophical, historical, psychological, and sociological accounts of science is live and important. Reductionist models presume that the sociological can be reduced to the cognitive or vice versa. Research on scientific inference has been accused of attempting reduction from the cognitive direction and assuming that social aspects of science can be reduced to psychological aspects. But I do not know of any researcher who has advocated this reductionist position. Perhaps there are still economists who think that macroeconomics can be reduced to microeconomics, but I know of no current advocate of the view that sociology can or should be reduced to psychology. Not only are social phenomena too complex to be reduced to psychological ones, but psychological explanations themselves must make reference to social factors. Slezak (1989) might be read as arguing that artificial intelligence can explain scientific discovery so that sociological explanations are redundant. But his position does not entirely reject sociological explanations, only the claims by some sociologists that scientific knowledge is able to explain everything.

In contrast, sociological reductionism has advocates. It surfaced in the 1930s in the Marxist history of science that overgeneralized Marx's statement that social existence determines consciousness. More recently, Collins (1990, p. 6) takes a sociological reductionist position when he claims that: "what we are as individuals is but a symptom of the groups in which the irreducible quantum of knowledge is located. Contrary to the usual reductionist model of the social sciences, it is the individual who is made of social groups."

What I call *residue* approaches do not claim to reduce the cognitive to the social or vice versa, but they nevertheless claim that one approach takes priority over the other. Laudan considers, but does not endorse, restricting the sociology of science by an *arationality assumption*: "The sociology of knowledge may step in to explain beliefs if and only if those beliefs cannot be explained in terms of their rational merits" (Laudan 1977, p. 202). This principle says that sociology is relevant only to the residue of scientific practice that remains after models of rationality have been applied. But I see no advance reason why in trying to understand science we should give special preference to explanations of belief change in terms of rationality. Instead, we should attempt to give the best explanation we can of particular scientific episodes, judging for each episode what factors were paramount.

Whereas the arationality principle sees the social as the residue of the cognitive, some sociologists see the cognitive as the residue of the social (Latour 1987, p. 256; Latour and Woolgar 1986, p. 280; Woolgar 1989, p. 217). Explanations in terms of cognitive capacities are to be resorted to only if the period of sociological investigation leaves anything to explain. In contrast, Bloor's (1991) most recent account of the "strong programme" in the sociology of science welcomes background theories of individual cognitive processes.

It is tempting to give a sociological explanation for the advocacy of reductionist and residue models. Arguments that one's own field is the main road to understanding of science can be viewed as tactics for increasing the influence and resources of researchers in that field. A more charitable interpretation of such arguments takes into account the frequent efficacy of single-mindedness as a research strategy. Sociologists can be seen as trying to push social explanations as far as possible to see how much they can accomplish, whereas psychologists and philosophers push a cognitive approach as far as possible. We could thus see sociological and psychological approaches as relatively autonomous from each other, overlapping occasionally to cooperate in explaining some developments in science while sometimes making competing explanations. This autonomy model of the psychology and sociology of science provides a reasonably accurate picture of the current state of science studies. By focusing on different aspects of science, researchers in different fields have increased the understanding of different contributors to the development of scientific knowledge. However, in the spirit of the Integrated Cognitive-Social Explanation Schema presented in chapter 1, I use the DAI perspective to go beyond an autonomy model without attempting to reduce in either direction or to relegate one approach to being the residue of the other.

My attempt to relate some of the social dimensions of science to cognition and computation raises important questions in the philosophy of social science regarding explanation. Methodological individualism is the doctrine that all attempts to explain social and individual phenomena must refer exclusively to facts about individuals (Lukes 1973). This doctrine has found most favor among conservative economists who contend that macroeconomic explanations that involve nations and organizations must ultimately yield to microeconomic explanations that involve decisions of individuals. According to methodological individualism, social explanations can and eventually should be reduced to psychological explanations. Viewing science as distributed computation does not, however, presuppose methodological individualism, for several reasons. First, in DAI, as in the analyses of sociologists such as Durkheim, there are facts that are irreducibly social. Second, psychological explanations are dependent on sociological explanations just as sociological explanations are dependent on psychological ones. Third, even explanations of individual computational psychology may need to be couched in social terms. Fourth, social phenomena are far too complex for us to expect a reduction of sociology to psychology to be tractable. Let us consider these reasons in more detail.

1. Durkheim, one of the founders of modern sociology, tried to distinguish social facts from ones that are only psychological. He wrote: "When I perform my duties as a brother, a husband or a citizen and carry out the commitments I have entered into, I fulfill obligations which are defined in law and custom and which are external to myself and my actions" (Durkheim 1982, p. 50). He argued that the compellingness of certain kinds of behavior and thinking derives from their external, social character. "What constitutes social facts are the beliefs, tendencies, and practices of the group taken collectively" (Durkheim 1982 p. 54) Mandelbaum characterizes "societal facts" more generally as "any facts concerning the forms of organization present in a society" (Mandelbaum 1973, p. 107). Does the view of science as distributed computation involve social facts in this sense? One might think that the organization of a computer network could be described in terms that are concerned only with the relations between individual processors. We can define the whole network by simply noting for each processor what other processors it is connected to. Such a characterization might work for simple computer networks, but it would clearly be inadequate for a scientific community that is viewed as a network of communicating computers. We can only understand why a cluster of scientists communicate intensely with each other by noting that the cluster is some particular kind of social organization: The scientists may be part of the same research group, teaching institution, or scientific organization. An account of why communication is asymmetric, with more information passing from one node to another than vice versa, often requires noting the differential social statusus of the scientists. Students usually learn more from professors than vice versa. Thus, although a DAI analysis can go some way to characterizing the communication structure of a scientific community, it does not attempt to eliminate social facts about its organization. To understand why there is a communication link between two scientists, we need to know that they belong to the same group, institution, or scientific society, so the DAI approach does not pretend to reduce these collectives to the individuals and their links.

2. Much of the plausibility of methodological individualism comes from the ontological point that societies consist of their members, although this does not imply that we can explain the operation of societies by attending only to the behavior of their members. Consider the explanation of why a particular scientist thinks and behaves in certain ways. I presume that the explanation will take the form of a description of the computational apparatus that produces the scientist's thinking, which includes a representation of what he or

she knows. Some of this knowledge will be about the world, and representation of it may suffice to explain much of the scientist's thinking, as when it is restricted to forming and evaluating hypotheses. But the scientist's thinking will often require the representation of social organizations, as in the following examples:

A. The scientist decides what funding agency to approach or how to frame planned research so it will be appealing to the agencies.

B. The scientist instead decides to pursue one project rather than another because it has greater potential for being appreciated by his or her academic department or research institution.

C. The scientist decides to submit a paper to a particular journal because it is widely read and respected by the field.

D. The scientist decides to attend a particular conference because relevant new work is likely to be presented there.

If we were building a simulation of the cognitive processes used by the scientist in decision making, we would therefore have to represent information about social entities such as agencies, departments, fields, and conferences. Thus, psychological explanations of scientist's thinking are in part sociological. My point here is supplemental to the one about social facts: A full model of science must take into account not only the ineliminable organization of science but also the mental representation of that organization by scientists.

3. Psychological explanations may turn out to be social in an additional sense. One of the leading figures in artificial intelligence, Marvin Minsky (1986), has contended that individual minds should be analyzed in terms of many smaller processes that can be conceptualized as "agents" organized in "societies." If Minsky's provocative but untested theory is correct, concepts drawn from sociology and distributed artificial intelligence will prove crucial for understanding the operations of individual minds.

4. Even if social phenomena could in principle be reduced to psychological ones, there are several technical reasons for doubting that the reduction would ever be carried out. First, cognitive phenomena may be indeterministic with ineliminably random elements. Some connectionist models for example, implement asynchronous updating of nodes by randomly choosing what node will next be updated. Hence, characterization of the thinking of individuals can be done only statistically, making it difficult to envision how operations of whole societies could be accounted for on the basis of the variable behavior of their members. Second, the combinatorics of describing the operation of societies in terms of their members are likely to make any reduction computationally intractable. If the operation and organization of a network of communicating scientists were made precise, it would probably be easy to show that the problem of predicting the overall behavior of the network from the behavior of

individual processors belongs to a large class of computational problems that require more time and storage space than any computer that could ever be built (Thagard 1993).

My third and final reason for doubting that the reduction of the social to the individual in computer networks will ever be practical derives from chaos theory. It is known that natural systems involving as few as three nonlinearly related independent variables can undergo chaotic behavior that is fully deterministic but utterly unpredictable, because minuscule differences in the initial conditions of the system generate exponentially diverging behavior. Even a simple damped and driven pendulum turns out to be subject to chaotic behavior, and more complex systems such as the weather have shown bounds to predictability. Huberman and Hogg (1987) have detected phase transitions in simple parallel computing networks. Similarly, it would be amazing if much more complex systems of interacting intelligent processors were not also subject to chaos, making explanation of the operation of whole networks in terms of their parts impracticable.

In sum, the point of conceiving of scientific communities as systems of distributed computation is not to reduce the sociological to the psychological but rather to increase coevolving understanding of societies and minds. This perspective is useful for considering important questions that concern group rationality and the division of cognitive labor.

RATIONALITY

According to the logical empiricist tradition, philosophical analyses that provide rational reconstructions of science should proceed without psychological taint. However, a psychological approach to science and epistemology is compatible with sufficiently complex models of rationality (see chapters 4 and 7 in this text, and Thagard 1988, 1992b). Principles of rationality are not to be derived a priori but should develop in interaction with increasing understanding of human cognitive processes. The cognitive approach to the study of science does not assume that psychological processes are rational, but it can assess the extent to which the various mental operations of scientists contribute to rationality. Similarly, social processes such as collaboration, the meeting of consensus panels, and Internet communication can be subjects for rational evaluation with respect to how well they further the epistemic and social goals of science (see chapters 11–13). Both psychological and sociological investigations can support the rationality of scientific practices from the cognitive (e.g., hypothesis evaluation) to the social (e.g., collaboration). We can also consider the relation between the rationality of individual scientists and the rationality of groups of scientists.

Sarkar (1983) raised the provocative possibility that group rationality in science is not merely the sum of individual rationality. If all scientists made identical judgments about the quality of available theories and the value of possible research programs, science would become homogeneous. Novel ideas and potentially acceptable new theories would never be developed sufficiently to the point where they would in fact become rationally acceptable by all. It was certainly fortunate that Marshall and Warren did not share the beliefs and conceptual systems of the gastroenterology establishment. Scientific revolutions are by no means instantaneous, and they often require a period of years for a new theory to be sufficiently developed that it poses a strong challenge to an entrenched view. Thagard (1988) suggested that viewing scientific communities as heterogeneous processors operating in parallel could provide a model of the division of labor that would enhance scientific progress. I conjectured that differences in motivation among scientists could lead them to work on different projects and thus provide better overall scientific progress than if everyone abided by identical standards of rationality. Kitcher (1993) used mathematics drawn from population biology to analyze how scientific progress may optimally require the division of cognitive labor and suggested that psychological and institutional factors that are often thought to be detrimental to cognitive progress might turn out to play a constructive role. Similarly, Hull (1989) considered how individual differences can contribute to the development of science viewed as a selection process. Solomon (1992) suggested how cognitive heuristics and biases can play an important role in decision making and promote the division of cognitive labor.

The social perspective that accompanies the view of a scientific community as a system for distributed computation provides a different view of the origin of the division of cognitive labor that seems necessary for rapid scientific progress. Differences in the motivation of individual scientists and their being subject to cognitive biases can undoubtedly lead them to pursue different projects, but the same result can also arise from the nature of distributed computation. Solomon suggests that in the development of geological theories, "different beliefs are largely explained at the level of individual cognition, as due to the heuristics of availability, representativeness, and salience, which lead to different results with different individual experience and prior belief, even when all the data are public knowledge" (Solomon 1992, p. 450). A DAI perspective makes it clear that we cannot expect all scientists in a field to be operating with the same information.

There are several impediments to the universal spread of information in a computational network. First, such networks may be sparsely connected, with only circuitous routes between two given processors. Thus, a theory or datum generated at one node is not immediately communicated to all other nodes. Sparseness of connectivity can be a function of national and institutional factors and of the psychological fact that no one can read everything or talk to everyone. Second, communication is asynchronous, with no overall "clock" governing the processing that occurs at each node. Some scientists may sit on new data, theories, or explanations for long periods before sending them along to others. Third, the overall process of transmission is slow. It can take months or years to publish results in a journal, and additional time may be required before even a habitual reader of the journal gets around to looking at it. Fourth, the overall process of transmission is incomplete. As we saw in the discussion of tacit knowledge, not everything that a scientist knows is communicated orally or in print to others, and natural language processing is such that scientists often fail to encode much of what they read for reasons that are independent of motivation and biases.

All these impediments contribute to the heterogeneousness of different nodes in the network of scientific computation. Not surprisingly, scientists who have received different information from the different groups with whom they communicate may tend to make different decisions. Individual scientists each start with a different stock of personal knowledge and experience: Even if they have exactly the same rational processes, we should expect them to have knowledge bases that do not completely converge because of the impossibility of perfect communication. One of the advantages of viewing science from the perspective of distributed artificial intelligence is that it becomes possible to imagine doing experiments to test the efficacy of various social strategies. As described in chapter 11, Clearwater et al. (1991) found that a group of cooperating agents engaged in problem solving can solve a task faster than either a single agent or the same group of agents working in isolation from each other. I look forward to further computational experiments that concern the efficacy of viewing science as a cooperative and competitive process.

REALISM

At the end of chapter 5, I argued that examination of the development of the bacterial theory of ulcers supports medical realism: the view that diseases and their causes are real and that scientific investigation can gain knowledge of them. In contrast, a recent social-historical treatment of the development of the genetic theory of cancer asserts: "I adhere to the basic assumption that the similarities [in practices] produced by oncogene researchers are the results of situated work and not of ontological reality" (Fujimura 1996, p. 216). Fujimura claims that oncogene research vindicates oncogene theory in the sense that it produced a scientific bandwagon in which many people, laboratories, and organizations committed their resources to this approach. Her sociological approach rules out any acknowledgment that cancer researchers in the 1980s converged on the oncogene theory in part because oncogenes exist and have the causal power to produce cancer. She approvingly quotes Hacking's (1992, p. 31) remark about laboratory science: "Our preserved theories and world fit together so snugly less because we have found how the world is than because we have tailored each to the other." Fujimura (1996, p. 13) espouses a kind of pragmatism in which "truth and knowledge are relative matters, malleable and dynamic."

Such pragmatism is implausible for the ulcers case, as well as for many other developments in medicine and science. It is incapable of explaining many aspects of scientific practice, such as the following:

1. The recalcitrance of experimentation: Researchers often obtain surprising results from their experiments, including undesired outcomes, such as when skeptics confirmed rather than refuted Marshall's claim that antibiotics cure ulcer.

2. The reliability of instruments: Microscopes and other instruments provide robust results across different social groups, as when the observation and culturing of *H. pylori* was replicated all over the world.

3. The causal efficacy of theory: Theories that are well supported by experiments often have profound technological and practical effects, as in the thousands of people who have already had ulcers cured by antibiotic treatment that presupposes the bacterial theory of ulcers.

4. The realist nature of scientific discourse: Scientists talk of discovering entities such as *H. pylori* and establishing causal relations, but the pragmatist must dismiss such discourse as epistemologically naive.

The epistemological naivete instead resides in academics who are so caught up in the social intricacies of scientific research that they (1) ignore the cognitive processes that enable scientists to assess the explanatory coherence of competing hypotheses and (2) underestimate the robustness of the physical processes that are involved in experiments. When Bishop and Weinberg (1996, p. 1) assert that causes of cancer act by damaging genes, they are relying on a wealth of experiments whose repeatability cannot be explained away as a bandwagon effect. Are scientists deluded in thinking that systematic observation, painstakingly controlled experiments, and rigorous hypothesis evaluation can teach us about the world? The delusion lies instead in those who think that science is just another semiotic exercise like literary criticism or fashion design.

It is unfortunate that medical research has not yielded general cures for cancer as it has for infectious diseases such as ulcers, but numerous novel treatment strategies are currently being investigated within the theoretical framework provided by the oncogene theory and other work in molecular biology (Israel 1996). The pragmatist must find it amazing that clever scientists with expensive laboratories and elaborate social relations have not been able to produce a cure for cancer. What has prevented the eruption of a scientific bandwagon that can alleviate the millions of deaths that occur from cancer and heart disease every year? For the medical realist, there is no mystery here—just an extraordinary difficult problem of understanding how the world works so that diseases can be dealt with more effectively.

In 1900, infectious diseases such as typhoid fever, measles, scarlet fever, diphtheria, pneumonia, and syphilis were major causes of death. Today, in economically advanced countries, deaths from these diseases are rare, with tuberculosis rates having dropped in the United States by a factor of more than two hundred. The preventive strategies (e.g., vaccination) and treatments (e.g., antibiotics) that contributed to these improvements make sense only if the germ theory of disease is understood as a realistic explanation of how micro-organisms make people sick. The medical bandwagon of the 1990s that saw gastroenterologists shift from skepticism about the bacterial theory of ulcers to its adoption and application makes sense only if we appreciate the reality of *H. pylori* bacteria and their causal relations with ulcers and antibiotics.

In social and cultural studies, antirealism is sometimes espoused as a politi-cal strategy intended to strip natural science of its epistemic authority to make room for an appreciation of other ways of knowing. But since the emergence of modern empirical science around the sixteenth century, no other mode of thinking and acting has even approximated science's ability to generate theoretical understanding and practical applications. Realism about entities, theories, and causes is an essential ingredient in understanding the growth of knowledge in science and medicine.

CONCLUSION

Socially and cognitively, science involves a tension between cooperation and competition, and researchers are only beginning to understand how social or-ganization can contribute to the overall goal of increasing scientific knowl-edge. But we can agree that science is social knowledge without neglecting the role of individual cognition in its development. By combining a computational understanding of individual cognition with an analysis of scientific communi-ties in terms of distributed computation, we can begin to see how sociological and psychological accounts of science can be integrated.

In the preface, I suggested that understanding science was like understand-ing disease: Both require attention to multiple interacting factors. The distrib-uted computing model of scientific research provides a way of integrating consideration of the cognitive processes of scientific researchers with the so-cial processes that enable them to communicate and collaborate. Chapters 11 to 13 showed that social processes can be subject to epistemic evaluation, just as much as cognitive processes. Although the emphasis in chapters 7 to 13 was on the psychological and the social, interactions with the world were an ongoing concern. Chapters 7 and 12 discussed the kinds of medical experiments that are most valuable for providing information about diseases and their causes. The point of using randomized clinical trials is to extract from the world maximally reliable information about treatments that will improve patients' health. Chapter 10 discussed conceptual change in terms of reference to the world as well as mental representation. Mind, society, and world all have figured in my picture of science.

I have tried in this book to give a broad, integrated, rational, and realist view of how science is conducted. The development and acceptance of the bacterial theory of ulcers provides a vivid illustration of the psychological, social, and physical processes that together enable researchers to understand the world. The growth of medical knowledge depends on the multiple interactions that constitute science as a complex system.

SUMMARY

The cognitive and social processes in science should not be viewed in isolation from each other but as part of a complex computational system that is analogous to those now being investigated in DAI. From this perspective, it is clear that the social does not reduce to the psychological, nor the psychological to the social. Scientific communities are systems in which the cognitive operations of an individual researcher feed into and respond to a large network of scientists. Construing science as distributed computing takes seriously the mental processes involved in the discovery and acceptance of theories as well as the social interactions among scientists. We can subject psychological and social processes to rational evaluation, and maintain the realist view that science tells us about a world that is independent of our minds and societies.

References

Ackermann, R. J. (1985). *Data, instruments, and theory*. Princeton, NJ: Princeton University Press.

Ahn, W., and Bailenson, J. (1996). Causal attribution as a search for underlying mechanism: An explanation of the conjunction fallacy and the discounting principle. *Cognitive Psychology, 31*, 82–123.

Ahn, W., Kalish, C. W., Medin, D. L., and Gelman, S. (1995). The role of covariation versus mechanism information in causal attribution. *Cognition, 54*, 299–352.

Anderson, J. R. (1983). *The architecture of cognition*. Cambridge, MA: Harvard University Press.

———. (1993). *Rules of the mind*. Hillsdale, NJ: Erlbaum.

Anderson, R. M., Schawatländer, B., McCutchan, F., and Hu, D. (1996). Implications of genetic variability in HIV for epidemiology and public health. *Lancet, 347*, 1778–1779.

Aronowitz, S. (1988). *Science as power: Discourse and ideology in modern society*. Minneapolis: University of Minnesota Press.

Barnes, B. (1985). *About science*. Oxford: Blackwell.

Barnes, B., Bloor, D., and Henry, J. (1996). *Scientific knowledge: A sociological analysis*. Chicago: University of Chicago Press.

Bartlett, J. G. (1996). Protease inhibitors for HIV infection. *Annals of Internal Medicine, 124*, 1086–1087.

Bell, D. S. (1995). *The doctor's guide to chronic fatigue syndrome*. Reading, MA: Addison-Wesley.

Berlinger, N. T. (1996). The breath of life. *Discover* (March), 102–104.

Biela, A. (1991). *Analogy in science*. Frankfurt: Peter Lang.

Bishop, J. M., and Weinberg, R. A. (Eds.). (1996). *Scientific American molecular oncology*. New York: Scientific American Books.

Blaser, M. J. (Ed.). (1989). *Campylobacter pylori in gastritis and peptic ulcer disease*. New York: Igaku-Shoin.

Bloor, D. (1991). *Knowledge and social imagery* (2nd ed.). Chicago: University of Chicago Press.

Bond, A., and Gasser, L. (Eds.). (1988). *Readings in distributed artificial intelligence*. San Mateo, CA: Morgan Kaufmann.

BonJour, L. (1985). *The structure of empirical knowledge*. Cambridge, MA: Harvard University Press.

Bradbury, S. (1968). *The microscope past and present*. Oxford: Pergamon.

Bradley, G. W. (1993). *Disease, diagnosis, and decisions*. Chichester, England: John Wiley & Sons.

Brock, T. D. (Ed.). (1961). *Milestones in microbiology*. Englewood Cliffs, NJ: Prentice-Hall.

———. (1988). *Robert Koch: A life in medicine and bacteriology*. Madison, WI: Science Tech Publishers.

Brody, H. (1996). Wired science. *Technology Review, 99*(October), 42–51.

Bromberger, S. (1992). *On what we know we don't know: Explanation, theory, linguistics, and how questions shape them.* Chicago: University of Chicago Press.

Brown, J. R. (Ed.). (1984). *Scientific rationality: The sociological turn.* Dordrecht, The Netherlands: Reidel.

———. (1989). *The rational and the social.* London: Routledge.

Brown, P., and Gajdusek, D. C. (1991). The human spongiform encephalopathies: Kuru, Creutzfeldt-Jakob disease, and the Gerstmann-Sträussler-Scheinker syndrome. In B. W. Chesebro (Ed.), *Transmissible spongiform encephalopathies: Scrapie, BSE, and related disorders* (pp. 1–20). Berlin: Springer-Verlag.

Buchwald, J. Z. (1992). Kinds and the wave theory of light. *Studies in History and Philosophy of Science, 23,* 39–74.

Bull, J. P. (1959). The historical development of clinical trials. *Journal of Chronic Diseases, 10,* 218–248.

Bulloch, W. (1979). *The history of bacteriology.* New York: Dover.

Bynum, W. F. (1993). Nosology. In W. F. Bynum and R. Porter (Eds.), *Companion encyclopedia of the history of medicine* (pp. 335–356). London: Routledge.

Callon, M. (1986). Some elements of a sociology of translation: Domestication of the scallops and the fisherman of St. Brieuc Bay. In J. Law (Ed.), *Power, action, and belief: A new sociology of knowledge* (pp. 196–229). London: Routledge and Kegan Paul.

Campbell, D. (1988). *Methodology and epistemology for social science: Selected papers.* Chicago: University of Chicago Press.

Caplan, A. L., Engelhardt, H. T., and McCartney, J. M. (Eds.). (1981). *Concepts of health and disease: Interdisciplinary perspectives.* Reading, MA: Addison-Wesley.

Carey, S. (1985). *Conceptual change in childhood.* Cambridge, MA: MIT Press/ Bradford Books.

———. (1992). The origin and evolution of everyday concepts. In R. N. Giere (Ed.), *Cognitive models of science* (pp. 89–128). Minneapolis: University of Minnesota Press.

Carpenter, K. J. (1986). *The history of scurvy and vitamin C.* Cambridge: Cambridge University Press.

Cartwright, N. (1989). *Nature's capacities and their measurement.* Oxford: Clarendon Press.

Chandrasekaran, B., Glasgow, J., and Narayanan, N.H.A.N. (Eds.). (1995). *Diagrammatic reasoning: Cognitive and computational perspectives.* Cambridge, MA: AAAI Press/MIT Press.

Cheng, P. W. (1997). From covariation to causation: A causal power theory. *Psychological Review, 104,* 367–405.

Chi, M. (1992). Conceptual change within and across ontological categories: Examples from learning and discovery in science. In R. Giere (Ed.), *Cognitive models of science, Minnesota studies in the philosophy of science* (pp. 129–186). Minneapolis: University of Minnesota Press.

Chinn, C. A., and Brewer, W. F. (1996). Mental models in data interpretation. *Philosophy of Science, 63*(proc. suppl.), S211–S219.

Churchland, P. (1989). *A neurocomputational perspective.* Cambridge, MA: MIT Press.

Clarfield, A. M., Kogan, S., Bergman, H., Shapiro, D. E., and Beaudet, M. P. (1996). Do consensus conferences influence their particpants? *Canadian Medical Association Journal, 154*, 331–336.

Clearwater, S., Huberman, B., and Hogg, T. (1991). Cooperative solution of constraint satisfaction problems. *Science, 254*, 1181–1183.

Coghlan, J. G., Gilligan, D., Humphries, H., McKenna, D., Dooley, C., Sweeney, E., Keane, C., and O'Morain, C. (1987). *Campylobacter pylori* and recurrence of duodenal ulcers—a 12-month follow-up study. *Lancet, 2*, 1109–1111.

Cohen, J. (1994). The Duesberg phenomenon. *Science, 266*, 1642–1644.

Collard, P. (1976). *The development of microbiology*. Cambridge: Cambridge University Press.

Collinge, J., and Palmer, M. S. (1992). Molecular genetics of inherited, sporadic, and iatrogenic prion disease. In S. B. Prusiner, J. Collinge, J. Powell, and B. Anderton (Eds.), *Prion diseases of humans and animals* (pp. 95–119). New York: Ellis Horwood.

Collins, H. (1985). *Changing order: Replication and induction in scientific practice*. London: Sage Publications.

———. (1990). *Artificial experts: Social knowledge and intelligent machines*. Cambridge, MA: MIT Press.

Comroe, J.H.J. (1977). *Retrospectroscope: Insights into medical discovery*. Menlo Park, CA: Von Gehr Press.

Conant, J. (1964). *Harvard case histories in experimental science*. Cambridge, MA: Harvard University Press.

Cover, T. L., and Blaser, M. J. (1992). *Helicobacter pylori* and gastroduodenal disease. *Annual Review of Medicine, 43*, 133–145.

Crane, D. (1972). *Invisible colleges: Diffusion of knowledge in scientific communities*. Chicago: University of Chicago Press.

Cutler, A. F., Havstad, S., Ma, C. K., Blaser, M. J., Perez-Perez, G. I., and Schubert, T. T. (1995). Accuracy of invasive and noninvasive tests to diagnose *Helicobacter pylori* infection. *Gastroenterology, 109*, 136–141.

Cziko, G. (1996). *Without miracles: Universal selection theory and the second Darwinian revolution*. Cambridge, MA: MIT Press.

D'Andrade, R. (1995). *The development of cognitive anthropology*. Cambridge: Cambridge University Press.

Dal Canto, M. C. (1991). Human and experimental spongiform encephalopathies: Recent progess in pathogenesis. *Italian Journal of Neurological Science, 12*, 147–153.

Darden, L. (1983). Artificial intelligence and philosophy of science: Reasoning by analogy in theory construction. In P. Asquith and T. Nickles (Eds.), *PSA 1982* (pp. 147–165). East Lansing, MI: Philosophy of Science Association.

Darden, L. (1991). *Theory change in science: Strategies from Mendelian genetics*. Oxford: Oxford University Press.

Darden, L., and Cain, J. (1989). Selection type theories. *Philosophy of Science, 56*, 106–129.

Darwin, C. (1958). *The autobiography of Charles Darwin and selected letters*. New York: Dover.

de Boer, W., Driessen, W., Jansz, A., and Tytgat, G. (1995). Effect of acid suppression on efficacy of treatment for *Helicobacter pylori* infection. *Lancet, 345*, 817–820.

Denissenko, M. F., Pao, A., Tang, M., and Pfeifer, G. P. (1996). Preferential formation of benzo[a]pyrene adducts at lung cancer mutational hotspots in P53. *Science, 274* 430–432.

Djerassi, C. (1989). *Cantor's dilemma.* New York: Doubleday.

Dobell, C. (1958). *Antony von Leeuwenhoek and his 'little animals.'* New York: Russell & Russell.

Donovan, A. (Ed.). (1988). *The chemical revolution: Essays in reinterpretation. Osiris,* 4(second series), entire issue.

Downes, S. M. (1993). Socializing naturalized philosophy of science. *Philosophy of Science, 60,* 452–468.

Dreyfus, H. L. (1992). *What computers still can't do* (3rd ed.). Cambridge, MA: MIT Press.

Duesberg, P. H. (1988). HIV is not the cause of AIDS. *Science, 241,* 514–517.

Dunbar, K. (1995). How scientists really reason: Scientific reasoning in real-world laboratories. In R. J. Sternberg and J. Davidson (Eds.), *Mechanisms of insight* (pp. 365–395). Cambridge, MA: MIT Press.

———. (1997). How scientists think: On-line creativity and conceptual change in science. In T. B. Ward, S. M. Smith, and J. Vaid (Eds.), *Creative thought: An investigation of conceptual structures and processes* (pp. 461–493). Washington, D.C.: American Psychological Association.

Durfee, E., Lesser, V., and Corkhill, D. (1989). Cooperative distributed problem solving. In A. Barr, P. Cohen, and E. Feigenbaum (Eds.), *The handbook of artificial intelligence. Vol. 4.* (pp. 83–147). Reading, MA: Addison-Wesley.

Durfee, E. H. (1992). What your computer really needs to know, you learned In kindergarten. In *Proceedings of the Tenth International Conference on Artificial Intelligence* (pp. 858–864). Menlo Park, CA: AAAI Press/The MIT Press.

Durkheim, E. (1982). *The rules of sociological method.* (Trans. W. Halls.) New York: Free Press.

Eells, E. (1991). *Probabilistic causality.* Cambridge: Cambridge University Press.

Eisenstein, E. L. (1979). *The printing press as an agent of change,* 2 vols. Cambridge: Cambridge University Press.

Eliasmith, C., and Thagard, P. (1997). Waves, particles, and explanatory coherence. *British Journal for the Philosophy of Science, 48,* 1–19.

Elwood, J. M. (1988). *Causal relationships in medicine.* Oxford: Oxford University Press.

EUROGAST Study Group (1993). An international association between *Helicobacter pylori* infection and gastric cancer. *Lancet, 341,* 1359–1362.

Evans, A. S. (1993). *Causation and disease: A chronological journey.* New York: Plenum.

Fekety, R. (1994). Infection and chronic fatigue syndrome. In S. E. Straus (Ed.), *Chronic fatigue syndrome* (pp. 101–179). New York: Marcel Dekker.

Fendrick, A. M., Hirth, R. A., and Chernew, M. E. (1996). Differences between generalist and specialist physicians regarding *Helicobacter pylori* and peptic ulcer disease. *American Journal of Gastroenterology, 91,* 1544–1548.

Forbes, G. M., Glaser, M. E., Cullen, D.J.E., Warren, J. R., Christianson, K. J., and Marshall, B. J. (1994). Duodenal ulcer treated with *Helicobacter pylori* eradication: Seven year follow-up. *Lancet, 342,* 258–260.

Forman, D., Newell, D. G., Fullerton, F., Yarnell, J. W., Stacey, A. R., Wald, N., and Sitas, F. (1991). Association between infection with *Helicobacter pylori* and risk of gastric cancer: Evidence from a prospective investigation. *British Medical Journal, 302*, 1302–1305.

Fracastorius, H. (1930). *Contagion, contagious diseases, and their treatment.* Trans. W. C. Wright. New York: G. P. Putnam's Sons.

Friedman, L. M., Furberg, C. D., and DeMets, D. L. (1981). *Fundamentals of clinical trials.* Boston: John Wright.

Fujimura, J. H. (1996). *Crafting science: A sociohistory of the quest for the genetics of cancer.* Cambridge, MA: Harvard University Press.

Fukuda, K., Straus, S. E., Hickie, I., Sharpe, M. C., Dobbins, J. G., and Komaroff, A. (1994). The chronic fatigue syndrome: A comprehensive approach to its definition and study. *Annals of Internal Medicine, 121*, 953–959.

Fung, W. P., Papadimitriou, J. M., and Matz, L. R. (1979). Endoscopic, histological, and ultrastructural correlations in chronic gastritis. *American Journal of Gastroenterology, 71*, 269–279.

Funk, C. (1912). The etiology of deficiency diseases. *Journal of State Medicine, 20*, 341–368.

Gajdusek, D. C., and Zigas, V. (1957). Degenerative disease of the central nervous system in New Guinea: The endemic occurrence of "kuru" in the native population. *New England Journal of Medicine, 257*, 974–978.

Gajdusek, D. C., Gibbs, C. J., and Alper, M. P. (1966). Experimental transmission of a kuru-like syndrome in chimpanzees. *Nature, 209*, 794–796.

Galison, P. (1987). *How experiments end.* Chicago: University of Chicago Press.

———. (1997). *Image and logic: A material culture of microphysics.* Chicago: University of Chicago Press.

Gallo, R. (1991). *Virus hunting.* New York: Basic Books.

Gallo, R. C., and Montagnier, L. (1989). The AIDS epidemic. In *The science of AIDS: Readings from Scientific American magazine* (pp. 1–11). New York: W. H. Freeman.

Gärdenfors, P. (1988). *Knowledge in flux.* Cambridge, MA: MIT Press/Bradford Books.

Gasser, L. (1991). Social conceptions of knowledge and action: DAI and open systems semantics. *Artificial Intelligence, 47*, 107–138.

Gentner, D., Brem, S., Ferguson, R., Wolff, P., Markman, A. B., and Forbus, K. (1997). Analogy and creativity in the works of Johannes Kepler. In T. B. Ward, S. M. Smith, and J. Vaid (Eds.), *Creative thought: An investigation of conceptual structures and processes* (pp. 403–459). Washington, DC: American Psychological Association.

Gick, M. L., and Holyoak, K. J. (1980). Analogical problem solving. *Cognitive Psychology, 12*, 306–355.

Giere, R. (1988). *Explaining science: A cognitive approach.* Chicago: University of Chicago Press.

———. (Ed.). (1992). *Cognitive models of science.* Minneapolis: University of Minnesota Press.

Giere, R. N. (1994). The cognitive structure of scientific theories. *Philosophy of Science, 61*, 276–296.

Glymour, C., Scheines, R., Spirtes, P., and Kelly, K. (1987). *Discovering causal structure.* Orlando, FL: Academic Press.

Goldman, A. (1986). *Epistemology and cognition.* Cambridge, MA: Harvard University Press.

Goldman, A. I. (1992). *Liaisons: Philosophy meets the cognitive and social sciences.* Cambridge, MA: MIT Press.

Gooding, D. (1990). *Experiment and the nature of meaning.* Dordrecht, The Netherlands: Kluwer.

Goodwin, C. S., Armstrong, J. A., Chilvers, T., Peters, M., Collins, M. D., Sly, L., McConnell, W., and Harper, W.E.S. (1989). Transfer of *Campylobacter pylori* and *Campylobacter mustelae* to *Helicobacter gen. nov.* as *Helicobacter pylori comb. nov.* and *Helicobacter mustelae comb. nov.,* respectively. *International Journal of Systematic Bacteriology, 39,* 397–405.

Goodwin, C. S., and Worsley, B. W. (1993). The *Helicobacter* genus: The history of *H. pylori* and taxonomy of current species. In C. S. Goodwin and B. W. Worsley (Eds.), Helicobacter pylori: *Biology and clinical practice* (pp. 1–13). Boca Raton, FL: CRC Press.

Grafe, A. (1991). *A history of experimental virology.* Trans. E. Reckendorf. Berlin: Springer-Verlag.

Graham, D. Y. (1989). *Campbylobacter pylori* and peptic ulcer disease. *Gastroenterology, 96,* 615–625.

———. (1991a). *Helicobacter pylori*: Its epidemiology and its role in duodenal ulcer disease. *Journal of Gastroenterology and Hepatology, 6,* 105–113.

———. (1991b). Present status of research and outlook for the future: What did we accomplish? In F. Halter, A. Garner, and G.N.J. Tytgat (Eds.), *Mechanisms of peptic ulcer healing* (pp. 303–309). Dordrecht, The Netherlands: Kluwer.

———. (1993). Treatment of peptic ulcers caused by *Helicobacter pylori. New England Journal of Medicine, 328,* 349–350.

———. (1995). *Helicobacter pylori*: Current status of diagnosis, therapy, pathophysiology, and thinking. In *Year book of medicine* (pp. xvii–xxxviii). St. Louis, MO: Mosby–Year Book.

———. (1996). Choosing the best anti–*Helicobacter pylori* therapy: Effect of antimicrobial resistance. *American Journal of Gastroenterology, 91,* 1072–1076.

Graham, D. Y., and Go, M. F. (1993). *Helicobacter pylori*: Current status. *Gastroenterology, 105,* 279–282.

Graham, D. Y., Klein, P. D., Evans, D. J., Jr., Evans, D. G., Alpert, L. C., Opekun, A. R., and Boutton, T. W. (1987). *Campylobacter pylori* detected non-invasively with the ^{13}C-urea breath test. *Lancet, 1,* 1174–1177.

Graham, D. Y., Lew, G. M., Klein, P. D., Evans, D. G., Evans, D. J., Saeed, Z. A., and Malaty, H. M. (1992). Effect of treatment of *Helicobacter pylori* infection on long-term recurrence of gastric or duodenal ulcer: A randomized, controlled study. *Annals of Internal Medicine, 116,* 705–708.

Graham, J. R. (1995). *Helicobacter pylori*: Human pathogen or simply an opportunist? *Lancet, 345,* 1095–1097.

Greenberg, D. L., and Root, R. K. (1995). Decision making by analogy. *New England Journal of Medicine, 332,* 592–596.

Grmek, M. D. (1981). L'invention de l'auscultation médiate. *Revue du palais de la découverte*(22), 107–116.

———. (1990). *History of AIDS.* Trans. R. C. Maulitz and J. Duffin, Princeton, NJ: Princeton University Press.

Guerlac, H. (1961). *Lavoisier—the crucial year*. Ithaca, NY: Cornell University Press.

Guyton de Morveau, L. B., Lavoisier, A. L., Berthollet, C. L., and de Fourcroy, A. F. (1787). *Méthode de nomenclature chimique*. Paris: Cuchet.

Hacking, I. (1983). *Representing and intervening*. Cambridge: Cambridge University Press.

———. (1992). The self-vindication of the laboratory sciences. In A. Pickering (Ed.), *Science as practice and culture* (pp. 29–64). Chicago: University of Chicago Press.

———. (1993). Working in a new world: The taxonomic solution. In P. Horwich (Ed.), *World changes: Thomas Kuhn and the nature of science* (pp. 275–310). Cambridge, MA: MIT Press.

Hadden, R. W. (1988). Social relations and the content of early modern science. *British Journal of Sociology*, *39*, 255–280.

Hadlow, W. J. (1959). Scrapie and kuru. *Lancet*, *2*, 289–290.

———. (1992). The scrapie-kuru connection: Recollections of how it came about. In S. B. Prusiner, J. Collinge, J. Powell, and B. Anderton (Eds.), *Prion diseases of humans and animals*. New York: Ellis Horwood.

Hardwig, J. (1985). Epistemic dependence. *Journal of Philosophy*, *82*, 335–349.

———. (1991). The role of trust in knowledge. *Journal of Philosophy*, *88*, 693–708.

Harman, G. (1986). *Change in view: Principles of reasoning*. Cambridge, MA: MIT Press/Bradford Books.

Harré, R., and Madden, E. (1975). *Causal powers*. Oxford: Blackwell.

Have, A.M.J.T., Kimsma, G. K., and Spicker, S. F. (Eds.). (1990). *The growth of medical knowledge*. Dordrecht,: The Netherlands: Kluwer.

Heidel, W. A. (1941). *Hippocratic medicine: Its spirit and method*. New York: Columbia University Press.

Hempel, C. G. (1965). *Aspects of scientific explanation*. New York: The Free Press.

Hennekens, C. H., and Buring, J. E. (1987). *Epidemiology in medicine*. Boston: Little, Brown.

Hentschel, E., Brandstätter, G., Dragosics, B., Hirschl, A. M., Nemec, H., Schütze, K., Taufer, M., and Wurzer, H. (1993). Effect of ranitidine and amoxicillin plus metronidazole on the eradication of *Helicobacter pylori* and the recurrence of duodenal ulcer. *New England Journal of Medicine*, *328*, 308–312.

Hewitt, C. (1991). Open information systems semantics for distributed artificial intelligence. *Artificial Intelligence*, *47*, 79–106.

Hintikka, J., and Vandamme, F. (Eds.). (1985). *Logic of discovery and logic of discourse*. New York: Plenum.

Hippocrates (1988). *Hippocrates. Vol. 5*. Trans. P. Cambridge, MA: Harvard University Press.

Hirschowitz, B. I. (1993). Development and application of endoscopy. *Gastroenterology*, *104*, 337–342.

Ho, D. D., Neumann, A. U., Perelson, A. S., Chen, W., Leonard, J. M., and Markowitz, M. (1995). Rapid turnover of plasma virions and CD4 lymphocytes in HIV-1 infection. *Science*, *373*, 123–126.

Holland, J. H. (1975). *Adaptation in natural and artificial systems*. Ann Arbor: University of Michigan Press.

Holland, J. H., Holyoak, K. J., Nisbett, R. E., and Thagard, P. R. (1986). *Induction: Processes of inference, learning, and discovery*. Cambridge, MA: MIT Press/Bradford Books.

Holmes, F. (1985). *Lavoisier and the chemistry of life.* Madison: University of Wisconsin Press.

Holyoak, K. J., and Spellman, B. A. (1993). Thinking. *Annual Review of Psychology,* *44,* 265–315.

Holyoak, K. J., and Thagard, P. (1989). Analogical mapping by constraint satisfaction. *Cognitive Science, 13,* 295–355.

———. (1995). *Mental leaps: Analogy in creative thought.* Cambridge, MA: MIT Press/Bradford Books.

Hopkins, H. H., and Kapany, N. S. (1954). A flexible fiberscope using static scanning. *Nature, 173,* 39–41.

Hosking, S. W., Ling, T.K.W., Chung, S. C., Cheng, A. F., and Sung, J. J. (1994). Duodenal ulcer healing by eradication of *Helicobacter pylori* without anti-acid treatment: Randomised controlled trial. *Lancet, 343,* 508–510.

Howson, C., and Urbach, P. (1989). *Scientific reasoning: The Bayesian tradition.* LaSalle, IL: Open Court.

Huberman, B, and Hogg, T.. (1987). Phase transitions in artificial intelligence systems. *Artificial Intelligence, 33,* 155–171.

Hudson, R. P. (1983). *Disease and its control: The shaping of modern thought.* Westport, CT: Greenwood.

Hughes, S. S. (1977). *The virus: A history of the concept.* London: Heinemann.

Hull, D. (1989). *Science as a process.* Chicago: University of Chicago Press.

Humphreys, P. (1989). *The chances of explanation.* Princeton, N.J.: Princeton University Press.

Hunt, R., Thomson, A.B.R., and Consensus Conference Participants (1998). Canadian *Helicobacter pylori* Consensus Conference. *Canadian Journal of Gastroenterology, 12,* 31–41.

Israel, M. A. (1996). Molecular genetics in the management of patients with cancer. In J. M. Bishop and R. A. Weinberg (Eds.), *Scientific American molecular oncology* (pp. 205–237). New York: Scientific American.

Iwasaki, Y., and Simon, H. (1994). Causality and model abstraction. *Artificial Intelligence, 67,* 143–194.

Janis, I. L. (1982). *Groupthink: Psychological studies of policy decisions and fiascos* (2nd ed.). Boston: Houghton Mifflin.

Johnson, H. (1996). *Osler's Web: Inside the labyrinth of the chronic fatigue syndrome epidemic.* New York: Crown.

Johnson-Laird, P. N., and Byrne, R. M. (1991). *Deduction.* Hillsdale, NJ: Lawrence Erlbaum Associates.

Kahneman, D., Slovic, P., and Tversky, A. (1982). *Judgment under uncertainty: Heuristics and biases.* New York: Cambridge University Press.

Kantorovich, A. (1993). *Scientific discovery: Logic and tinkering.* Albany: State University of New York Press.

Keil, F. (1989). *Concepts, kinds, and cognitive development.* Cambridge, MA: MIT Press/Bradford Books.

Kelley, H. H. (1972). Causal schemata and the attribution process. In E. E. Jones, D. E. Kanouse, H. H. Kelley, R. E. Nisbett, S. Valins, and B. Weiner (Eds.), *Attribution: Perceiving the causes of behavior.* Morristown, NJ: General Learning Press.

Kettler, B., and Darden, L. (1993). Protein sequencing experiment planning using analogy. In L. Hunter (Ed.), *Artificial intelligence and molecular biology* (pp. 216–224). Menlo Park, CA: AAAI Press.

Kim, K. (1994). *Explaining scientific consensus: The case of Mendelian genetics*. New York: Guilford.

King, L. S. (1982). *Medical thinking: A historical preface*. Princeton, NJ: Princeton University Press.

Kiple, K. F. (Ed.). (1993). *The Cambridge world history of disease*. Cambridge: Cambridge University Press.

Kitcher, P. (1981). Explanatory unification. *Philosophy of Science, 48*, 507–531.

———. (1989). Explanatory unification and the causal structure of the world. In P. Kitcher and W. C. Salmon (Eds.), *Scientific explanation* (pp. 410–505). Minneapolis: University of Minnesota Press.

———. (1993). *The advancement of science*. Oxford: Oxford University Press.

Klahr, D., and Dunbar, K. (1988). Dual space search during scientific reasoning. *Cognitive Science, 12*, 1–48.

Kleiner, S. A. (1993). *The logic of discovery: A theory of the rationality of scientific research*. Dordrecht, The Netherlands: Kluwer.

Kolodner, J. (1993). *Case-based reasoning*. San Mateo, CA: Morgan Kaufmann.

Kornfeld, W., and Hewitt, C. (1981). The scientific community metaphor. *IEEE Transactions on Systems Man and Cybernetics, SMC-11*, 24–33.

Koslowski, B. (1996). *Theory and evidence: The development of scientific reasoning*. Cambridge, MA: MIT Press.

Koton, P. (1988). Reasoning about evidence in causal explanations. *Proceedings of the Seventh National Conference on Artificial Intelligence* (pp. 256–261). Cambridge, MA: MIT Press.

Koza, J. R. (1992). *Genetic programming*. Cambridge, MA: MIT Press.

Kuhn, T. (1970). *Structure of scientific revolutions* (2nd ed.). Chicago: University of Chicago Press.

Kuhn, T. S. (1993). Afterwords. In P. Horwich (Ed.), *World changes: Thomas Kuhn and the nature of science* (pp. 311–341). Cambridge, MA: MIT Press.

Kunda, Z. (1990). The case for motivated inference. *Psychological Bulletin, 108*, 480–498.

Kunda, Z., Miller, D. T., and Claire, T. (1990). Combining social concepts: The role of causal reasoning. *Cognitive Science, 14*, 551–577.

Kunda, Z., and Thagard, P. (1996). Forming impressions from stereotypes, traits, and behaviors: A parallel-constraint-satisfaction theory. *Psychological Review, 103*, 284–308.

Laennec, R. (1962). *A treatise on the diseases of the chest*. Trans. J. Forbes. New York: Hafner.

LaFollette, H., and Shanks, N. (1995). Two models of models in biomedical research. *Philosophical Quarterly, 45*, 141–160.

LaFollette, M. C. (1992). *Stealing into print: Fraud, plagiarism, and misconduct in scientific publishing*. Berkeley: University of California Press.

Langley, P. (1996). *Elements of machine learning*. San Francisco: Morgan Kaufmann.

Langley, P., and Jones, R. (1988). A computational model of scientific insight. In R. Sternberg (Ed.), *The nature of creativity: Contemporary psychological perspectives*. (pp. 177–201). Cambridge: Cambridge University Press.

Langley, P., Simon, H., Bradshaw, G., and Zytkow, J. (1987). *Scientific discovery.* Cambridge, MA: MIT Press/Bradford Books.

Latour, B. (1987). *Science in action: How to follow scientists and engineers through society.* Cambridge, MA: Harvard University Press.

———. (1988). *The pasteurization of France.* Trans. A. Sheridan and J. Law. Cambridge, MA: Harvard University Press.

Latour, B., and Woolgar, S. (1986). *Laboratory life: The construction of scientific facts.* Princeton, NJ: Princeton University Press.

Laudan, L. (1977). *Progress and its problems.* Berkeley: University of California Press.

Lauer, T. W., Peacock, E., and Graesser, A. C. (Eds.). (1992). *Questions and information systems.* Hillsdale, NJ: Erlbaum.

Leake, D. B. (1992). *Evaluating explanations: A content theory.* Hillsdale, NJ: Erlbaum

Leatherdale, W. H. (1974). *The role of analogy, model, and metaphor in science.* Amsterdam: North-Holland.

Lechevalier, H. A., and Solotorovsky, M. (1974). *Three centuries of microbiology.* New York: Dover.

Lehrer, K. (1990). *Theory of knowledge.* Boulder, CO: Westview.

Lenat, D., and Guha, R. (1990). *Building large knowledge-based systems.* Reading, MA: Addison-Wesley.

Levi, I. (1991). *The fixation of belief and its undoing.* Cambridge: Cambridge University Press.

Levin, A. (1984). Venel, Lavoiser, Fourcroy, Cabanis, and the idea of scientific revolution. *History of Science, 22,* 303–320.

Lind, J. (1953). *Lind's treatise on scurvy.* Edinburgh: Edinburgh University Press.

Linné, C. v. (1956). *Systema naturae.* London: British Museum of Natural History.

Lloyd, G.E.R. (Ed.). (1978). *Hippocratic writings.* London: Penguin.

Longino, H. (1990). *Science as social knowledge: Values and objectivity in scientific inquiry.* Princeton, NJ: Princeton University Press.

Lukes, S. (1973). Methodological individualism reconsidered. In A. Ryan (Ed.), *The philosophy of social explanation.* (pp. 119–129). Oxford: Oxford University Press.

Mackworth, A. (1993). On seeing robots. In A. Basu and X. Li (Eds.), *Computer vision: Systems, theory, and applications* (pp. 1–13). Singapore: World Scientific.

Magner, L. M. (1992). *A history of medicine.* New York: Marcel Dekker.

Malfertheiner, P., Mégraud, F., O'Morain, C., Bell, D., Bianchi Porro, G., Deltenre, M., Forman, D., Gasbarrini, G., Jaup, B., Misiewicz, J. J., Pajares, J., Quina, M., and Rauws, E. (1997). Current European concepts in the management of *Helicobacter pylori* infection—the Maastricht consensus report. *European Journal of Gastroenterology and Hepatology, 9,* 1–2.

Mandelbaum, M. (1973). Societal facts. In A. Ryan (Ed.), *The philosophy of social explanation* (pp. 105–118). Oxford: Oxford University Press.

Marshall, B. J. (1989). History of the discovery of *C. pylori.* In M. J. Blaser (Ed.), Campylobacter pylori in gastritis and peptic ulcer disease (pp. 7–22). New York: Igaku-Shoin.

———. (1994). *Helicobacter pylori. American Journal of Gastroenterology, 89*(8 suppl.), S116–S128.

Marshall, B. J., Armstrong, J. A., McGechie, D. B., and Clancy, R. J. (1985). Attempt to fulfil Koch's postulates for pyloric *Campbylobacter. Medical Journal of Australia, 142,* 436–439.

Marshall, B. J., Goodwin, C. S., Warren, J. R., Murray, R., Blincow, E. D., Blackbourn, S. J., Phillips, M., Waters, T. E., and Sanderson, C. R. (1988). Prospective double-blind trial of duodenal ulcer relapse after eradication of *Campylobacter pylori. Lancet, 2,* 1437–1441.

Marshall, B. J., Plankey, M. W., Hoffman, S. R., Boyd, C. L., Dye, K. R., Frierson, H. F., Guerrant, R. L., and McCallum, R. W. (1991). A 20-minute breath test for *Helicobacter pylori. American Journal of Gastroenterology, 86,* 438–445.

Marshall, B. J., and Warren, J. R. (1984). Unidentified curved bacilli in the stomach of patients with gastritis and peptic ulceration. *Lancet, 1,* 1311–1315.

Mathews, J. D., Glasse, R., and Lindenbaum, S. (1968). Kuru and cannibalism. *Lancet, 2*(7565), 449–452.

Mayo, D. (1996). *Error and the growth of experimental knowledge.* Chicago: University of Chicago Press.

McCann, H. (1978). *Chemistry transformed: The paradigmatic shift from phlogiston to oxygen.* Norwood, NJ: Ablex.

McCollum, E. V. (1957). *A history of nutrition.* Boston: Houghton Mifflin.

McEvoy, J. G. (1988). Continuity and discontinuity in the Chemical Revolution. *Osiris, 4,* 195–213.

McKusick, V. A., and Francomano, C. A. (Eds.). (1994). *Mendelian inheritance in man: A catalog of human genes and genetic disorders* (11th ed.). Baltimore: Johns Hopkins University Press.

Medin, D. L. (1989). Concepts and conceptual structure. *American Psychologist, 44,* 1469–1481.

Merton, R. K. (1973). *The sociology of science: Theoretical and empirical investigations.* Chicago: University of Chicago Press.

Michela, J. L., and Wood, J. V. (1986). Causal attributions in health and illness. In P. C. Kendall (Ed.), *Advances in cognitive-behavioral research and therapy. Vol. 5* (pp. 179–235). New York: Academic Press.

Middleton, R. G. (1997). Prostate cancer: Are we screening and treating too much? *Annals of Internal Medicine, 126,* 465–467.

Millgram, E., and Thagard, P. (1996). Deliberative coherence. *Synthese, 108,* 63–88.

Minsky, M. (1986). *The society of mind.* New York: Simon & Schuster.

Mitchell, T. (1997). *Machine learning.* New York: McGraw-Hill.

Monmaney, T. (1993). Marshall's hunch. *New Yorker,* September 20, 64–72.

Moravec, H. (1988). *Mind children: The future of robot and human intelligence.* Cambridge, MA: Cambridge University Press.

Muhlestein, J. B. (1997). The link between *Chlamydia pneumoniae* and atherosclerosis. *Infections in Medicine* [Internet version on Medscape], *14,* 380–392.

Munnangi, S., and Sonnenberg, A. (1997). Time trends of physician visits and treatment patterns of peptic ulcer disease in the United States. *Archives of Internal Medicine, 157,* 1489–1494.

Murphy, G., and Medin, D. (1985). The role of theories in conceptual coherence. *Psychological Review, 92,* 289–316.

Murray, P. R., Kobayaki, G. S., Pfaller, M. A., and Rosenthal, K. S. (1994). *Medical microbiology* (2nd ed.). St. Louis: Mosby.

National Institutes of Health Consensus Development Panel (1994). *Helicobacter pylori* in peptic ulcer disease. *Journal of the American Medical Association, 272,* 65–69.

Nersessian, N. (1989). Conceptual change in science and in science education. *Synthese, 80*, 163–183.

———. (1992). How do scientists think? Capturing the dynamics of conceptual change in science. In R. Giere (Ed.), *Cognitive models of science* (pp. 3–44). Minneapolis: University of Minnesota Press.

Newell, A. (1990). *Unified theories of cognition.* Cambridge, MA: Harvard University Press.

Newell, A., and Simon, H. A. (1972). *Human problem solving.* Englewood Cliffs, NJ: Prentice-Hall.

Nowak, G., and Thagard, P. (1992a). Copernicus, Ptolemy, and explanatory coherence. In R. Giere (Ed.), *Cognitive models of science*, (pp. 274–309). Minneapolis: University of Minnesota Press.

———. (1992b). Newton, Descartes, and explanatory coherence. In R. Duschl and R. Hamilton (Eds.), *Philosophy of science, cognitive psychology and educational theory and practice.* (pp. 69–115). Albany: State University of New York Press.

Nuland, S. B. (1988). *Doctors: The biography of medicine.* New York: Knopf.

Nutton, V. (1990). The reception of Fracastoro's theory of contagion: The seed that fell among thorns? *Osiris, 6* (second series), 196–234.

O'Brien, B., Goeree, R., Mohamed, H., and Hunt, R. (1996). Cost-effectiveness of *Helicobacter pylori* eradication for the long-term management of duodenal ulcer in Canada. *Archives of Internal Medicine, 155*, 1958–1964.

O'Hare, G.M.P., and Jennings, N. R. (Eds.). (1996). *Foundations of distributed artificial intelligence.* New York: John Wiley & Sons.

Olbe, L., Hamlet, A., Dalenbäck, J., and Fändriks, L. (1996). A mechanism by which *Helicobacter pylori* infection of the antrum contributes to the development of duodenal ulcer. *Gastroenterology, 110*, 1386–1394.

Pasteur, L. (1922). *Oeuvres.* Vol. 2. Paris: Masson.

Pearl, J. (1988). *Probabilistic reasoning in intelligent systems.* San Mateo, CA: Morgan Kaufman.

Peng, Y., and Reggia, J. (1990). *Abductive inference models for diagnostic problem solving.* New York: Springer-Verlag.

Perrin, C. E. (1987). Revolution or reform: The chemical revolution and eighteenth century concepts of scientific change. *History of Science, 25*, 395–423.

———. (1988). The chemical revolution: Shifts in guiding assumptions. In A. Donovan, L. Laudan, and R. Laudan (Eds.), *Scrutinizing science: Empirical studies of scientific change* (pp. 105–124). Dordrecht, The Netherlands: Kluwer.

Peterson, W. L. (1991). *Helicobacter pylori* and peptic ulcer disease. *New England Journal of Medicine, 324*, 1043–1048.

Peura, D. A. et. al. (in press). Report of the international update conference on *Helicobacter pylori. Gastroenterology.*

Pickering, A. (1992). From science as knowledge to science as practice. In A. Pickering (Ed.), *Science as practice and culture* (pp. 1–26). Chicago: University of Chicago Press.

———. (1995). *The mangle of practice: Time, agency, and science.* Chicago: University of Chicago Press.

Popper, K. (1959). *The logic of scientific discovery.* London: Hutchinson.

Proctor, R. N. (1995). *Cancer wars: How politics shapes what we know and don't know about cancer.* New York: Basic Books.

Prusiner, S. B. (1982). Novel proteinaceous infectious particles cause scrapie. *Science*, *216*, 136–144.

———. (Ed.). (1996). *Prions, prions, prions*. Berlin: Springer-Verlag.

Prusiner, S. B., Collinge, J., Powell, J., and Anderton, B. (Eds.). (1992). *Prion diseases of humans and animals*. New York: Ellis Horwood.

Rabinow, P. (1996). *Making PCR*. Chicago: University of Chicago Press.

Ram, A. (1991). A theory of questions and question asking. *Journal of the Learning Sciences*, *1*, 273–318.

Rauws, E.A.J., and Tytgat, G.N.J. (1990). Cure of duodenal ulcer with eradication of *Helicobacter pylori*. *Lancet*, *335*, 1233–1235.

Read, S., and Marcus-Newhall, A. (1993). The role of explanatory coherence in the construction of social explanations. *Journal of Personality and Social Psychology*, *65*, 429–447.

Renehan, E. J. (1996). *Science on the Web: 500 of the most essential science Web sites*. New York: Copernicus.

Reznek, L. (1987). *The nature of disease*. London: Routledge and Kegan Paul.

Rhodes, R. (1997). *Deadly feasts*. New York: Simon & Schuster.

Roberts, R. M. (1989). *Serendipity: Accidental discoveries in science*. New York: John Wiley & Sons.

Rohmer, R. G. (1991). The scrapie virus: "A virus by any other name." In B. W. Chesebro (Ed.), *Transmissible spongiform encephalopathies: Scrapie, BSE, and related disorders* (pp. 195–232). Berlin: Springer-Verlag.

Root-Bernstein, R. S. (1993). *Rethinking AIDS: The tragic cost of premature consensus*. New York: Free Press.

Ross, A. (Ed.). (1996). *Science wars*. Durham, NC: Duke University Press.

Rubenstein, E. (1994). Preface. In P. Leder, D. A. Clayton, and E. Rubenstein (Eds.), *Scientific American introduction to molecular medicine* (pp. vii-viii). New York: Scientific American.

Rumelhart, D. E., and McClelland, J. L. (Eds.). (1986). *Parallel distributed processing: Explorations in the microstructure of cognition*. Cambridge, MA: MIT Press/ Bradford Books.

Sackett, D. L., Rosenberg, W. M., Gray, J. A., Haynes, R. B., and Richardson, W. S. (1996). Evidence-based medicine: What it is and what it isn't. *British Medical Journal*, *312*, 71–72.

Salmon, W. (1984). *Scientific explanation and the causal structure of the world*. Princeton, NJ: Princeton University Press.

Sarkar, H. (1983). *A theory of method*. Berkeley: University of California Press.

Schaffner, K. F. (1993). *Discovery and explanation in biology and medicine*. Chicago: University of Chicago Press.

Schank, P., and Ranney, M. (1992). Assessing explanatory coherence: A new method for integrating verbal data with models of on-line belief revision. In *Proceedings of the Fourteenth Annual Conference of the Cognitive Science Society* (pp. 599–604). Hillsdale, NJ: Erlbaum.

Schank, R. C. (1986). *Explanation patterns: Understanding mechanically and creatively*. Hillsdale, NJ: Erlbaum.

Schunn, C. D., and Klahr, D. (1995). A 4-space model of scientific discovery. In J. D. Moore and J. F. Lehman (Eds.), *Proceedings of the Seventeenth Annual Conference of the Cognitive Science Society* (pp. 106–111). Mahwah, NJ: Erlbaum.

Schunn, C. D., Okada, T., and Crowley, K. (1995). Is cognitive science truly interdisciplinary? The case of interdisciplinary collaborations. In J. D. Moore and J. F. Lehman (Eds.), *Proceedings of the Seventeenth Annual Conference of the Cognitive Science Society* (pp. 100–105). Mahwah, NJ: Erlbaum.

Shafer, G. (1996). *The art of causal conjecture.* Cambridge, MA: MIT Press.

Shryock, R. H. (1969). *The development of modern medicine.* New York: Hafner.

Silverstein, A. M. (1989). *A history of immunology.* San Diego: Academic Press.

Simon, H. A., and Lea, G. (1974). Problem solving and rule induction: A unified view. In L. W. Gregg (Ed.), *Knowledge and cognition.* Hillsdale, NJ: Erlbaum.

Sinclair, W. J. (1909). *Semmelweiss: His life and his doctrine.* Manchester, England: Manchester University Press.

Skelton, J. A., and Croyle, R. T. (Eds.). (1991). *Mental representation in health and illness.* New York: Springer-Verlag.

Slezak, P. (1989). Scientific discovery by computer as empirical refutation of the strong programme. *Social Studies of Science, 19,* 563–600.

Slotta, J. D., Chi, M.T.H., and Joram, E. (1996). Assessing students' misclassifications of physics concepts: An ontological basis for conceptual change. *Cognition and Instruction, 13,* 373–400.

Smith, E. (1989). Concepts and induction. In M. Posner (Ed.), *Foundations of cognitive science* (pp. 501–526). Cambridge, MA: MIT Press.

Smith, E., and Medin, D. (1981). *Categories and concepts.* Cambridge, MA: Harvard University Press.

Solomon, M. (1992). Scientific rationality and human reasoning. *Philosophy of Science, 59,* 439–455.

———. (1994). Social empiricism. *Nous, 28,* 325–343.

Steer, H. W., and Colin-Jones, D. G. (1975). Mucosal changes in gastric ulceration and their response to carbenoxolone sodium. *Gut, 16,* 590–597.

Strachan, T., and Read, A. P. (1996). *Human molecular genetics.* New York: BIOS Scientific.

Straus, S. E. (Ed.). (1994). *Chronic fatigue syndrome.* New York: Marcel Dekker.

Sulloway, F. J. (1996). *Born to rebel: Birth order, family dynamics, and creative lives.* New York: Pantheon Books.

Suppes, P. (1970). *Probabilistic theory of causality.* Atlantic Highlands, NJ: Humanities Press.

Susser, M. (1973). *Causal thinking in the health sciences.* New York: Oxford University Press.

Suzuki, D. (1995). Ulcer wars [transcript of broadcast on CBC television]. *The Nature of Things* [originally produced by British Broadcasting Corporation].

Taubes, G. (1996). Science journals go wired. *Science, 271,* 764.

Temkin, O. (1973). Health and disease. In P. P. Wiener (Ed.), *Dictionary of the history of ideas* (pp. 395–407). New York: Charles Scribner's Sons.

———. (1977). *The double face of Janus.* Baltimore: Johns Hopkins University Press.

Thagard, P. (1988). *Computational philosophy of science.* Cambridge, MA: MIT Press/ Bradford Books.

———. (1992a). Adversarial problem solving: Modelling an opponent using explanatory coherence. *Cognitive Science, 16,* 123–149.

———.(1992b). *Conceptual revolutions.* Princeton, NJ: Princeton University Press.

————. (1993). Computational tractability and conceptual coherence: Why do computer scientists believe that P ≠ NP? *Canadian Journal of Philosophy, 23,* 349–364.

————.(1996). *Mind: Introduction to cognitive science.* Cambridge, MA: MIT Press.

————. (in press). Probabilistic networks and explanatory coherence. In P. O'Rorke and G. Luger (Eds.), *Computing explanations: AI perspectives on abduction.* Menlo Park, CA: AAAI Press.

Thagard, P., and Millgram, E. (1995). Inference to the best plan: A coherence theory of decision. In A. Ram and D. B. Leake (Eds.), *Goal-driven learning* (pp. 439–454). Cambridge, MA: MIT Press.

Thagard, P., and Verbeurgt, K. (1998). Coherence as constraint satisfaction. *Cognitive Science, 22,* 1–24.

Thomson, T. (1813). Biographical account of M. Lavoisier. *Annals of Philosophy, 2,* 81–92.

Tosteson, D. C., Adelstein, S. J., and Carver, S. T. (Eds.). (1994). *New pathways to medical education: Learning to learn at Harvard Medical School.* Cambridge, MA: Harvard University Press.

Vallery-Radot, R. (1926). *The life of Pasteur.* Trans. R. L. Devonshire. Garden City, NY: Doubleday.

van Fraassen, B. (1980). *The scientific image.* Oxford: Clarendon Press.

Warren, J. R., and Marshall, B. J. (1983). Unidentified curved bacilli on gastric epithelium in active chronic gastritis. *Lancet 1,* 1273–1275.

Wasserman, S., and Faust, K. (1994). *Social network analysis: Methods and applications.* Cambridge: Cambridge University Press.

Weinberg, R. A. (1996). *Racing to the beginning of the road: The search for the origin of cancer.* New York: Harmony Books.

Wessely, S. (1994). The history of chronic fatigue syndrome. In S. E. Straus (Ed.), *Chronic fatigue syndrome* (pp. 3–44). New York: Marcel Dekker.

Wittgenstein, L. (1956). *Remarks on the foundations of mathematics.* Oxford: Blackwell.

Woolgar, S. (1988). *Science: The very idea.* Chichester, England: Ellis Horwood.

————. (1989). Representation, cognition, and self: What hope for an integration of psychology and philosophy? In S. Fuller, M. De Mey, T. Shinn, and S. Woolgar (Eds.), *The cognitive turn: Sociological and psychological perspectives on science* (pp. 210–223). Dordrecht, The Netherlands: Kluwer.

Wyngaarden, J. B., Smith, L. H., and Bennett, J. C. (Eds.). (1992). *Cecil textbook of medicine* (19th ed.). Philadelphia: W. B. Saunders.

Zamir, M. (1996). Secrets of the heart. *The Sciences*(September/October), 26–31.

Index

Index